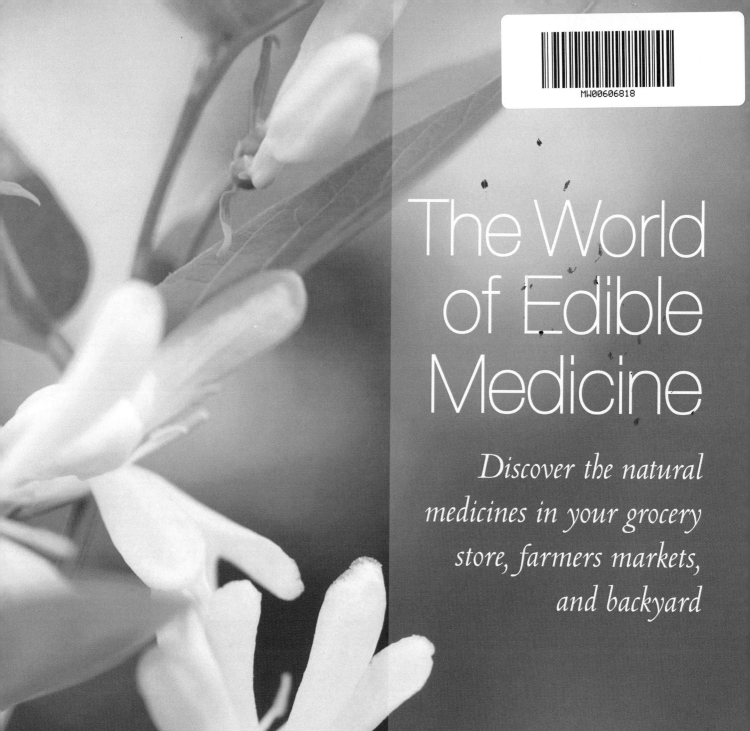

The World of Edible Medicine

Discover the natural medicines in your grocery store, farmers markets, and backyard

Dr. Barbara Custer, O.M.D.

Printed in the United States of America
ISBN 978-0-692-42805-4

Cover Design: *Diane Dias* | **Book Design:** *Jessica Gray, Diane Dias, Wesley Emblidge*

Special thanks to Holly Morrow, Ursula Kauth, Ruby Valentine, Lisa Martinez, Raina Williams, Wesley Emblidge, Kyle Dang, Jessica Gray, Micheala Bagley, and Diane Dias for their hard work and dedication. A big thank you to all the wonderful people who made this book possible.

Contents

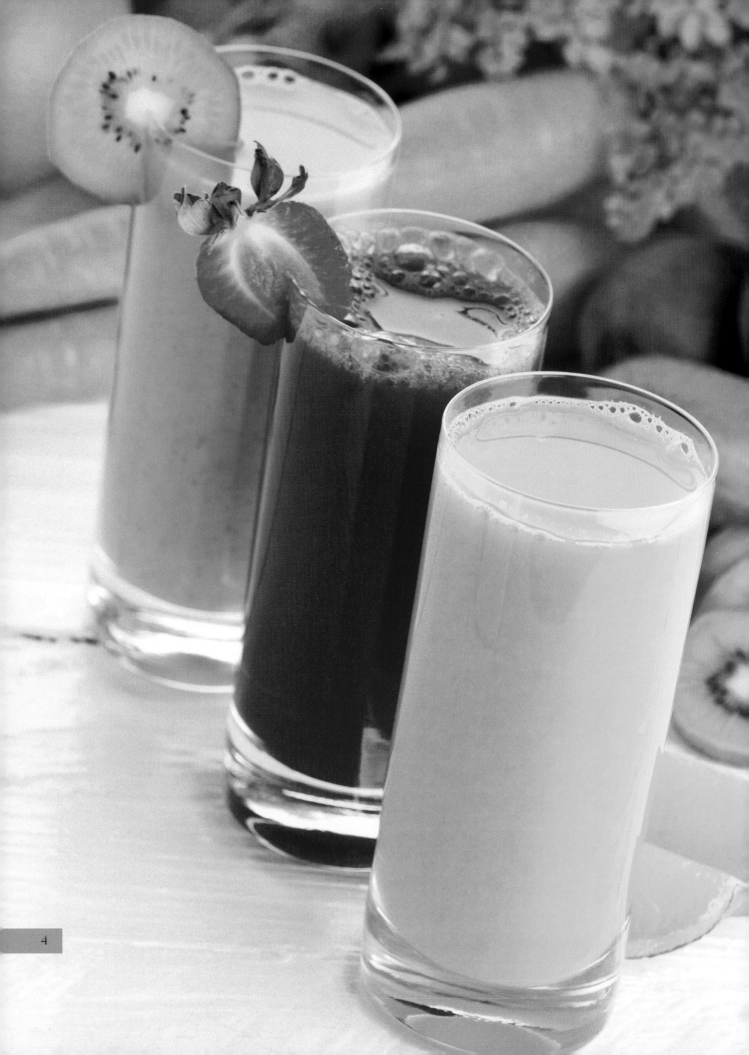

Preface

I have been asked over the years how I got involved in such an unconventional profession as Oriental Medicine. My journey into this fascinating medical system began with a prophetic dream about being a doctor in the Orient and an unforgettable love story. At the time of the dream, I was finishing college. I graduated with a B.A. in Studio Art, so practicing medicine was the furthest thing from my mind. The dream seemed very real but I dismissed it as irrelevant to what I was doing at the time or wanted to do in the future.

That summer I took a job in the mountains teaching swimming at an international students camp run by the University of California, Berkeley. The camp cook was a tall 6'2" man who looked like a Chinese movie star straight out of a Kung Fu movie. Not only was he gorgeous, he was also a self-taught gourmet chef.

The Asian connection was beginning. Together we made bok choy with sautéed mushrooms and oyster sauce. Pot stickers filled with fresh zucchini, ginger, and garlic. Spicy Szechwan eggplant. Barbecued Chinese-style chicken with grilled salt and pepper prawns. There were no hotdogs and s'mores that summer! I was learning how to cook amazing food and was falling crazy in love.

After the summer was over, my boyfriend and I moved to Berkeley. He had just completed college there and loved the area. In the late 1970s, Berkeley was a Mecca for everything new, unusual, different, and progressive. After a year together, my Chinese movie star boyfriend with his gorgeous satin skin began to develop psoriasis, a serious skin disease. He decided to try a natural treatment protocol for this problem. He did this by taking Chinese herbal medicine, having acupuncture treatments, and becoming a vegetarian. After his skin condition was successfully cured, I became more and more fascinated by the power of this type of medicine. I studied vegetarian cooking and took small classes in Oriental Medicine in San Francisco.

I continued my studies in Japan and the U.S. In 1983, I got my license to practice Oriental Medicine in

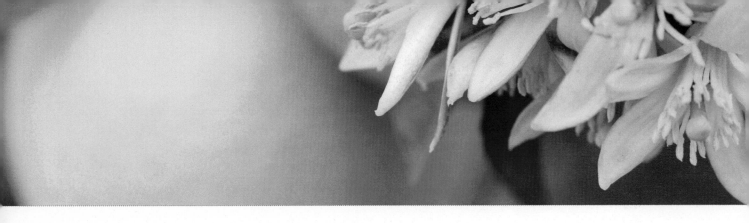

the United States. Even after studying and practicing Oriental Medicine for almost 30 years, I'm still fascinated by the power of this medicine. This form of medicine amazes me in ways that I can't comprehend with my rational Western mind.

Over the years of practicing, I have treated patients with diseases with scary titles, such as "Graves disease," "Hashimoto's," and "diabetes," using acupuncture, herbal medicine, diet, and lifestyle changes. This type of treatment is an effective way to get off medication and reverse disease patterns. I have seen older women get pregnant naturally and children with symptoms of ADD become focused and relaxed. What continues to fascinate me about this medical system is the way it can reverse disease and reduce or eliminate dependence on Western drugs.

I currently reside and practice in Mill Valley, California. I create individualized, Optimum Health and Wellness Programs for my clients, using Western medical testing and natural treatment protocols. I specialize in

endocrinology, the study of hormones. I use Western medical testing to decide what type of natural treatment protocols will be the most effective. The Western medical testing gives a directional guide on what the body is doing and the retesting shows if we have obtained the desired results.

Diet is an important foundation for this type of medicine. Over the years, I have also studied nutrition and different types of diets. Last year, I presented the first in a series of classes, called "Food Is Medicine." In the class we explored the medicinal properties of everyday healthy foods and new ways to prepare foods to make them exciting and delicious.

My goal is to use this book as a fun teaching tool to educate people about the importance of using food as their most basic medicine. I am currently incorporating cleanses and detox programs into my practice. These programs use fresh juices, Chinese herbal medicine, and natural supplements. So enjoy making food fun, exciting, delicious, and rejuvenating!

Introduction

As a society, we share a concern for the health and well-being of our children and all living things on Earth. We are just beginning to become aware of how to take care of our health. Diet is the most basic component of creating a state of optimum health. The vital nutrients in food produce the body's internal biochemistry, which then can directly affect our health and sense of well-being. Understanding the medicinal properties and health benefits of fruits, vegetables, medicinal flowers, culinary herbs, and spices can help us make more healthy choices.

Elaborate cuisines with specific food preparations come to us from all over the world. Every culture has certain foods that are eaten for health as well as ceremonial purposes. Some of the oldest and most elaborate texts come from Egypt, Greece, Iran, India, and China. These ancient texts, dating back more than 3,000 years, are some of the earliest documents we have about medicine, botany, and philosophy. Chinese medicine and Ayurvedic medicine include the most elaborate systems of diet and herbs used for the treatment of specific symptoms and illnesses. Many of these traditional herbal formulas and dietary recommendations continue to be used by Chinese and Ayurvedic doctors today.

Even today, cultures from around the globe still have unique foods and herbs that are considered "health foods." These foods are central to their diet, and are unique to the nutritional map of that specific culture.

Some examples of these traditional foods are: soybeans, tofu, seaweed, and green tea from Japan. Lemon grass tea, cilantro, and coconut milk from Thailand. Olive oil, yogurt, and goat cheese from Greece. Peppers, hot sauce, and hibiscus flower tea from the Latin American countries. Ginger, garlic, and jasmine flower tea from China. The World Health Organization estimates that 70% to 80% of the world's population currently uses herbs, spices, and foods as natural plant-based medicine.

From the plant kingdom comes the world of herbal and culinary medicine. Natural medicine practitioners

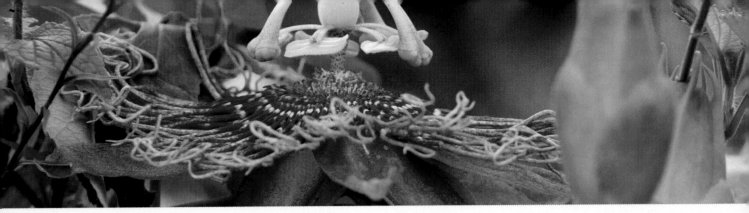

from around the world use concentrated plant extracts, high-dosed vitamins and minerals, and diet to rebalance the body and reverse disease patterns. Hippocrates, the famous Greek physician who is considered the father of Western medicine wrote, "Our food should be our medicine and our medicine should be our food."

There are over 20,000 natural chemical compounds that have been identified from plants. Concentrated amounts of organic chemical compounds derived from plants can produce a "medicine-like" effect in the body. For instance, high doses of vitamin C, derived from rose hips, have been proven to reduce inflammation and joint pain and to boost immune response. Concentrated honeysuckle flower extract reduces strep and staph bacteria, producing a natural antibiotic effect. Valerian root and passionflower extracts have a sedating effect on the nervous system and are used to treat anxiety and insomnia. Red Korean ginseng is known to boost adrenal

and testosterone hormones, promoting energy and elevating mood.

There are many benefits to using plant extracts and making health-oriented diet changes. Natural plant-derived extracts can help to reverse disease symptoms, have few side effects, and are nontoxic to the body.

If we want to eat for health, we need to know what we are eating and why it is good for us. With this understanding we can make more conscious, healthy, diet choices to use "food as medicine."

The foods that we are eating every day have so many natural vitamins, minerals, and phytochemicals that have been scientifically studied and have proven medicinal effects. Below are just some of the important natural chemicals found in the rainbow-colored fruits and vegetables.

Blue and purple fruits and vegetables derive their color from plant pigment called anthocyanin, a powerful antioxidant. Antioxidants are used by the body to reverse damage to cells caused by the effect of free radicals and radiation.

Green fruits and vegetables derive their color from chlorophyll and isothiocyanates. These natural chemicals stimulate liver enzymes that assist the body's ability to remove potentially carcinogenic compounds. Indoles are a naturally occurring plant chemical found in broccoli, kale, cabbage, and other cruciferous vegetables. They are being studied for their effect on inhibiting some types of tumor growth.

Red fruits and vegetables derive their color from lycopene, another powerful antioxidant. In a Mayo Clinic study, researchers found that high intake of lycopene-containing foods produced high lycopene serum levels in the blood. This plant compound has been proven to reverse damage to the cell walls of the heart and has been shown to reverse some types of macular degeneration.

Orange and yellow fruits and vegetables contain varying amounts of antioxidants such as vitamins C and A, as well as carotenoids and bioflavonoids. These natural chemicals are important for improving vision, increasing immune response, and enhancing collagen production.

The China Study is a book written to study the effects of diet, and is the largest and most comprehensive study of human nutrition ever conducted. It was launched via a partnership among Cornell University, Oxford University, and the Chinese Academy of Preventative Medicine. This study researched more than 8,000 statistically significant associations between lifestyle and diet. The results showed that people who ate the most animal proteins had the most chronic and degenerative disease symptoms. The people who ate the most plant-based foods were the healthiest and had the least chronic and degenerative diseases.

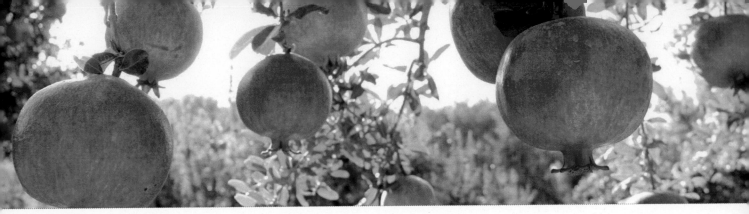

Dr. Caldwell Esselstyn, M.D., a physician and researcher at the Cleveland Clinic in Ohio, treated patients with established coronary heart disease with an organic foods and plant-based diet. Not only did this stop the progression of disease, 70% of patients saw a reversal of clogged arteries in the heart.

Dr. Dean Ornish, of Sausalito, California, a graduate of Harvard Medical School, completed a similar study with consistent results. His current research also showed that comprehensive lifestyle and plant-based diet changed gene expression, "turning on" disease-preventing genes and "turning off" genes that promote cancer and heart disease. This exciting finding means that we may have the possibility to stop disease patterns that seem to be hard-wired in our DNA.

With chronic and serious diseases on the rise in this country we must make our health and the health of our family and friends a priority. Healthy lifestyle changes such as diet and exercise have been proven to reverse disease patterns as well as be our best preventative medicine.

Fresh organic fruits and vegetables are delicious and offer us infinite varieties of colors, textures, aromas, and tastes. Fruits, vegetables, spices, and herbs found in our farmers markets and health food stores and grown in our gardens can not only change our health and vitality, but can also potentially reverse disease.

Cooking and making healthy, delicious food is a fun way to be with our friends and family, and it also establishes one of the most important things we can do for our health.

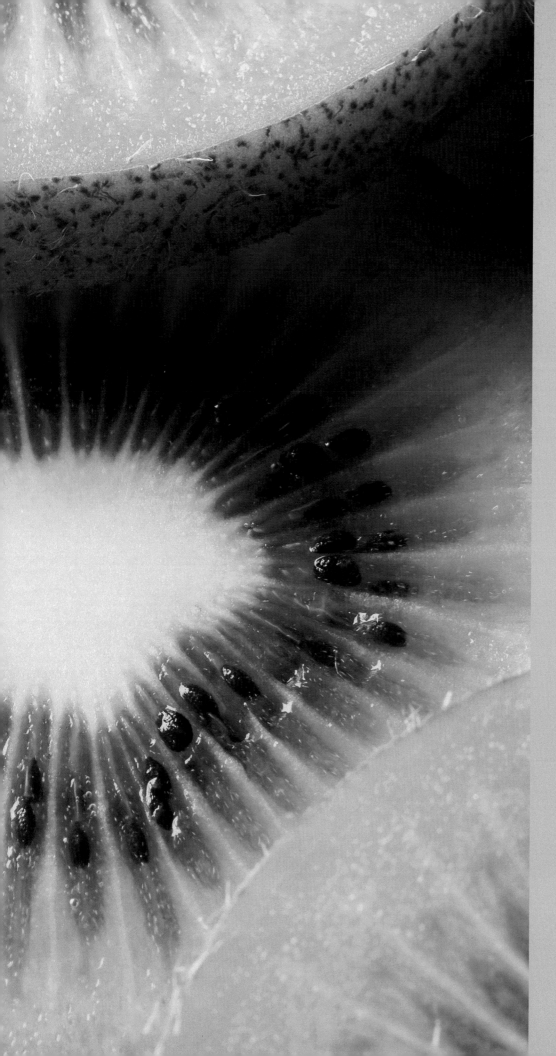

"I finally realized that being grateful to my body was key to giving more love to myself."
— *Oprah Winfrey*

Oprah Winfrey is an influential TV host, producer, and actress. She uses her influence to create awareness for healthy living, combating relevant social issues, and more.

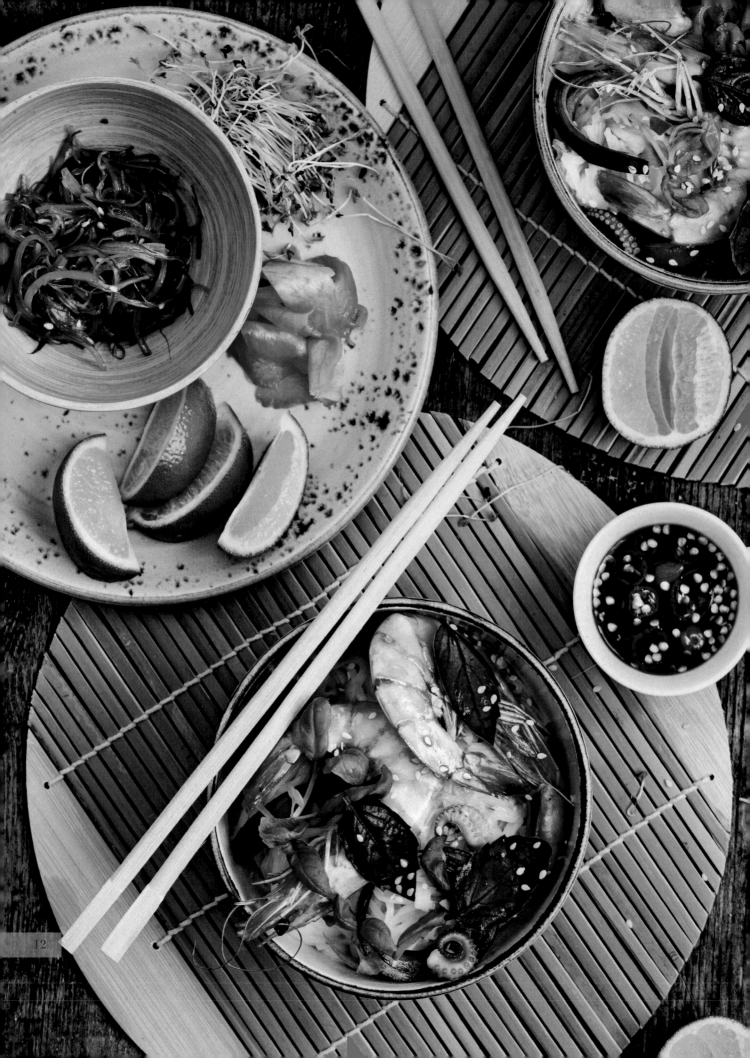

Eating for Pleasure, Health, & Fun

Understanding the medicinal properties and health benefits of fruits, vegetables, medicinal flowers, culinary herbs, and spices can give us the opportunity to make healthy choices that will greatly enhance our well-being. Some of the latest scientific research shows that plant-based diets can not only help to produce a state of optimal health, but have also shown the capability of being able to reverse disease patterns.

Ancient medicinal texts dating back more than 3,000 years have shown that this is not a new way of thinking. Texts from Egypt, Greece, Iran, India, and China are some of the earliest writings about medicine, botany, and philosophy. In these medicinal texts, diet and the use of medicinal plants were used for treatment of specific symptoms and illnesses.

Now science and modern medicine are beginning to prove the claims made by these ancient texts. Today diet and lifestyle are considered some of the most important ingredients for health. Natural medicine practitioners from around the world use diet, medicinal plant extracts, and high-dose vitamins and minerals to rebalance the body and reverse disease patterns. Start today by eating lots of bright-colored fruits and vegetables, making healthy choices, and enjoying a long, healthy, and prosperous life.

Hippocrates, a famous Greek physician who is considered the father of Western medicine, wrote: "Our food should be our medicine and our medicine should be our food."

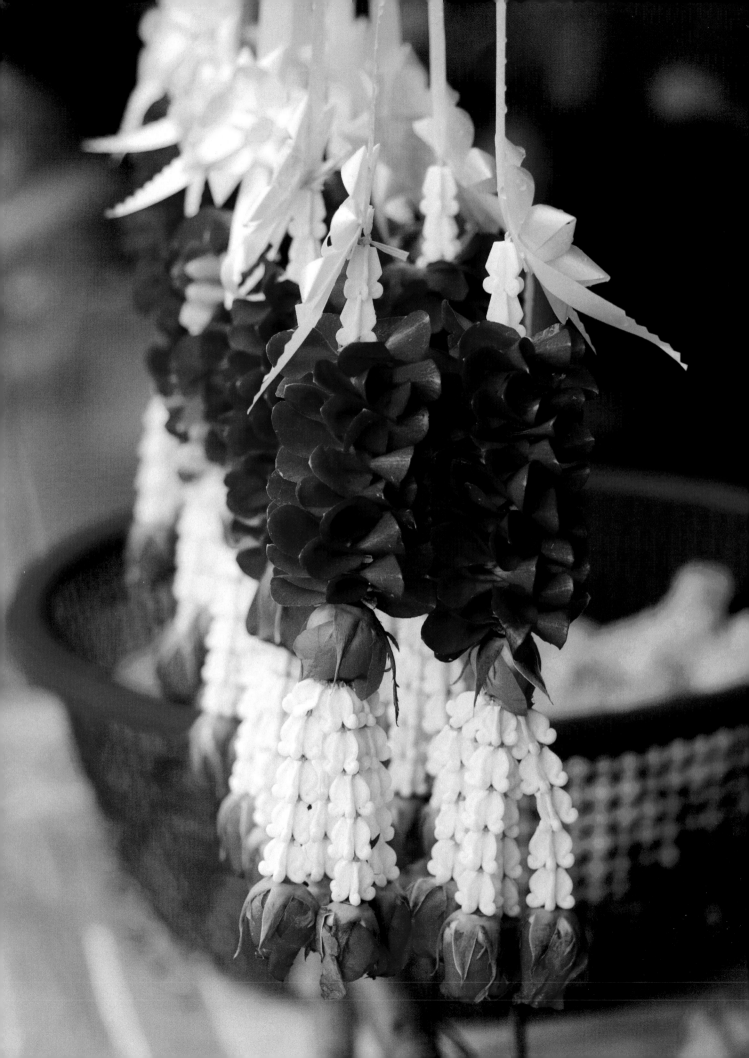

flowers: ancient medicines

Medicinal Flowers

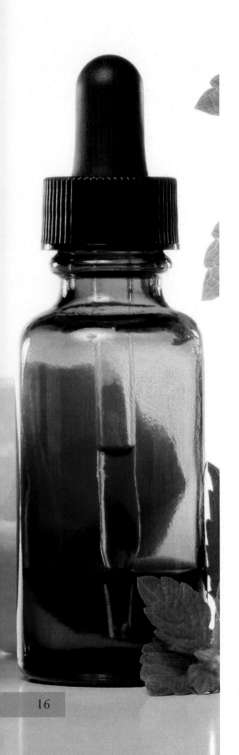

Flowers have always been revered for their beauty and held us captive with their mesmerizing array of scents, patterns, shapes, and colors. Roses, lilies, and gardenias are just some of the flowers with intoxicating fragrances. Distilled essences of gardenia, tuberose, and jasmine are some of the most common flowers used in perfumes and in many cosmetics. The essential oils of flowers have been used and treasured by all cultures and have created multi-million-dollar perfume industries.

Flowers are not only famous for their beauty, they are also some of the most important medicinal plants used for herbal medicines and teas. All cultures around the world use different medicinal flowers as medicines. Lilac flowers are used in herbal formulas to reduce fevers. Hibiscus flowers and rose hips are high in natural vitamin C. Morning glory flowers are used as natural laxatives. Plum blossom flowers are used in Chinese medicine as a natural treatment for intestinal bacteria and parasites. Valerian flowers and roots are used to calm the nerves and help with sleep.

The flowers mentioned in this section are just some of the important ones used in Chinese herbal medicine. Flowers can be used fresh or dried, or made into concentrated liquid extracts, powders, tinctures, and pill form. Many of the traditional formulas used in Chinese herbal medicine date back to *The Yellow Emperor's Classic of Medicine,* of 240 B.C.

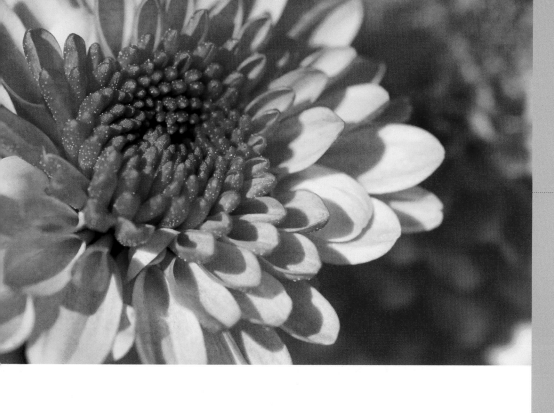

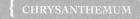

Chrysanthemum flowers, also known as mums, are native to China. They grow in many beautiful colors varying from white and red to pale chartreuse. They are commonly found at most local flower shops.

According to Chinese *Feng Shui*, this flower is symbolic of a balanced life. Drinking water infused with the flowers' essence is believed to bring good luck and immortality. Chrysanthemum flower tea is used to reduce high blood pressure, relieve tension headaches, ease flu symptoms, and lower fever. Chrysanthemum flower tea is served throughout Asia as an iced tea to cool the blood and reduce the effects of summer heat in the body.

The dried flowers are available at most Asian grocery stores and tea shops. The flowers make a beautiful tea. They unfold as the boiling water reconstitutes them to their original size and float to the surface of the cup. The next time you have a headache, try steeping a few dried flowers in hot water for 10 minutes and add honey to taste. In Asia, this flower tea is considered nature's aspirin in a cup.

Flowers are some of the most important plants in the world of natural herbal medicine. Many different types of flowers are used to treat symptoms from the common cold to insomnia.

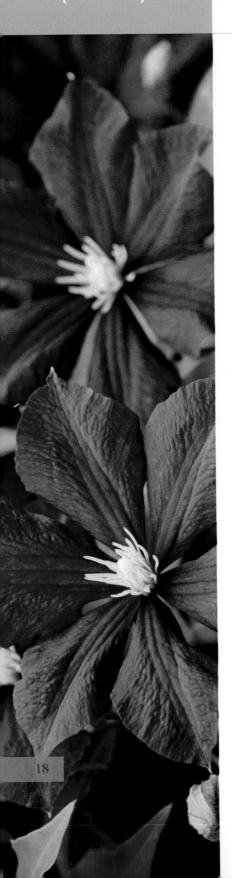

clematis & gardenia

Clematis is a beautiful climbing perennial shrub, part of the buttercup family. This family of flowers has approximately 350 different species that are common to North America and Asia. Seven species are used for their medicinal properties in Chinese medicine.

The most common flowers seen in North America are the beautiful vine-like variety, which have big, light purple flowers. The flowers can be three to four inches in diameter. In the 17th century, this stunning flower became a very popular decorative plant in Japanese gardens and can still be seen on Japanese flower motifs in paintings, ceramics, and textiles.

In Chinese medicine, clematis is used to treat pain, especially in the joints and connective tissues, such as arthritis and bursitis. The medicinal property of this plant works by creating blood circulation and helping to reduce inflammation and pain. Clematis flower works a lot like aspirin and ibuprofen, without the side effects. It is one of the most important medicinal herbs used to treat back pain.

This flower is not used alone, but together with other herbs. A famous Chinese formula that is used for alleviating the pain of arthritis is a combination of clematis and stephania. This formula is available through health care practitioners only.

The databases of the United States Department of Agriculture list over 200 species of gardenia flowers that have medicinal properties.

Gardenia is known for its beautiful white symmetrical blossoms and intoxicating scent. Originally found only in China and Japan, today gardenias are grown all over the world.

In Tahiti and Hawaii, the flowers are still worn to indicate a woman's marital status. If the flower is worn on the left ear it means that she is married. If the flower is worn on the right ear it means the woman is available and looking.

The databases from the United States Department of Agriculture list over 200 species of gardenia that have medicinal properties. In Chinese herbal medicine, gardenia is used to treat many different types of infections, due to its cooling effect on the blood.

Gardenia is an important medicinal flower used to treat bladder infections. When used together with chrysanthemum flower it has been shown to be an effective natural treatment for lowering high cholesterol.

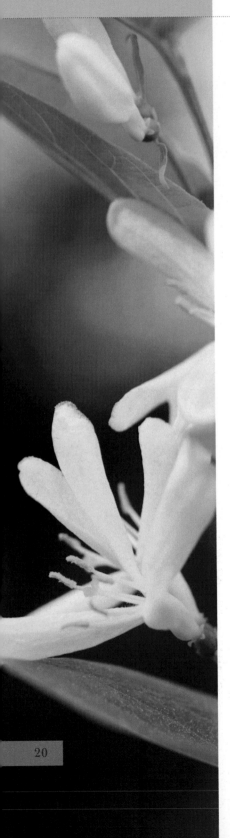

honeysuckle & jasmine

Honeysuckle is a flower native to East Asia. This fragrant and beautiful flower is a vine that grows profusely in many climates. The entire plant is used for medicinal purposes.

The honeysuckle flower has been called the "flower of love" because the blossoms look like two intertwined lovers. European legend says that if you bring honeysuckle flowers into your home there will be a wedding within a year. While this flower is famous for romance, it is equally famous for its culinary and medicinal purposes. The flower is edible and often used in Europe as a decoration for pastries. Many different products are made with honeysuckle flowers such as honeysuckle sorbet, wine, and jelly.

Honeysuckle flower has been proven to have natural antibiotic and antifungal effects. This is one of the most important flowers used in Chinese formulas to treat fever, colds, sore throats, and bronchitis.

At the first signs of a cold or flu, try using a famous Chinese herbal formula called *Yin Qiao*. This cold and flu remedy is available at most health food stores, herb shops, and health care practitioners.

Jasmine is one of the most prized flowers in Asia and the Middle East. It is revered not only for its intoxicating scent but also for its invaluable medicinal properties. Jasmine flowers are used in Asia and India for special occasions and ceremonies because of their beautiful scent. The essential oils of this flower are commonly used as a base for expensive perfumes and skin care products.

Recent research has validated the health benefits of jasmine. An extensive study conducted at Kyoto University in Japan found that this flower has a naturally sedative effect on the nervous system. The research showed jasmine flower extract to be beneficial in helping to relieve symptoms of anxiety, heart palpitations, and insomnia.

All jasmine tea is not created equal. Most commercial jasmine tea is usually mixed with green or black tea. This will not produce the same calming effects that pure jasmine flowers will, because of the high caffeine content in green and black teas. In health food stores and fine tea shops, you can buy dried jasmine flower buds. This tea is delicious prepared hot or iced; just add a little natural sweetener.

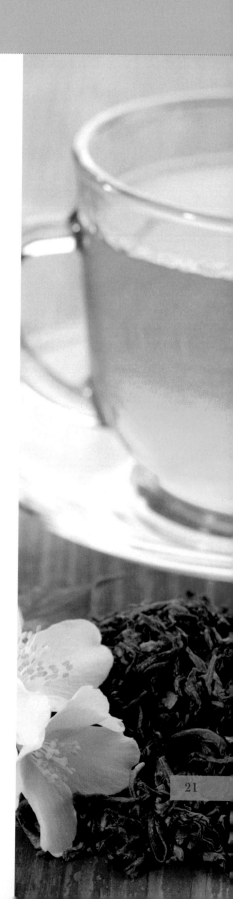

21

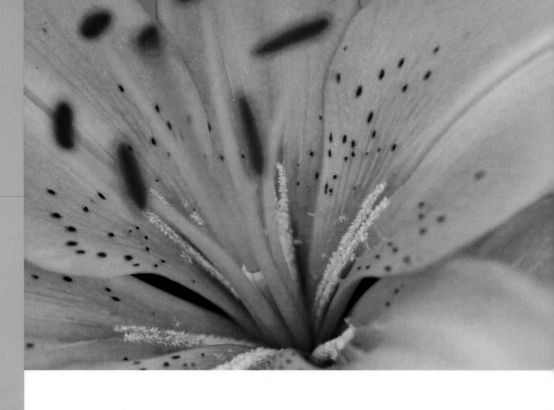

The bulbs of the tiger lily are used as food and medicine in the Americas and Asia. Considered a delicacy, the starchy bulb tastes similar to potatoes, and has been farmed in China for centuries.

Lilies have been cultivated as an ornamental plant and used as an herbal medicine for centuries. There are many varieties of lilies, found in all different shapes, colors, and sizes. The white Easter lily, the Casablanca lily, and the stargazer lily are the most common ornamental lilies. The orange tiger lily is the plant that is used as an herbal medicine.

In China, the bulbs are used in soups and in stir-fry vegetable dishes as they have a potato-like texture and taste. This plant is also written about in old European texts where the leaves and roots were used to make ointments and salves for the treatment of skin infections, rashes, and hives.

The bulbs of the orange tiger lily are used in traditional Chinese herbal medicine formulas. Dried lily bulbs are known for their analgesic properties. They are used to moisten the lungs, stop dry coughs, treat sore throats, and help relieve the tight chest and wheezing common to asthma.

lily & lotus

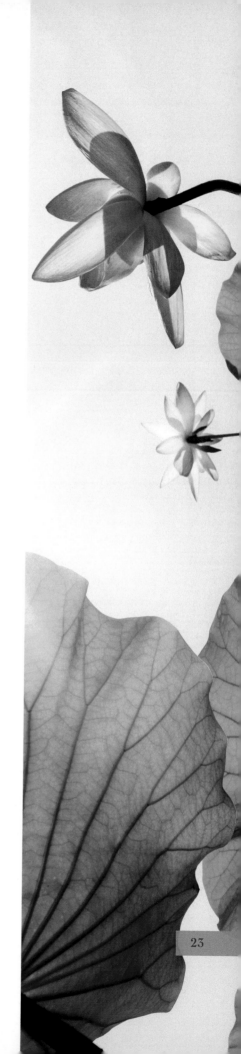

Lotus is the national flower of Egypt, India, and Vietnam. All the parts of this plant, including the flower, seeds, stems, and roots, are used for medicine, food, and teas.

In Buddhist tradition, this flower is revered because it represents the evolution of the human soul. This plant grows in very murky waters and blooms into a magnificent flower symbolizing the possibility for personal transformation within a person's lifetime.

The lotus root is a delicious vegetable that has the taste of a potato and crispiness of celery. The root is typically used like a potato. It is usually added to soups and can also be made into cold summer salads. Moon cakes, a special Chinese pastry, are made from lotus root and red bean paste. They are eaten at the fall equinox in September and used to celebrate the fall harvest.

The powdered lotus root, readily found in Chinese grocery stores, makes a delicious hot tea with honey. It is a very effective natural remedy used for strengthening the lungs and relieving dry, lingering coughs after a cold or flu.

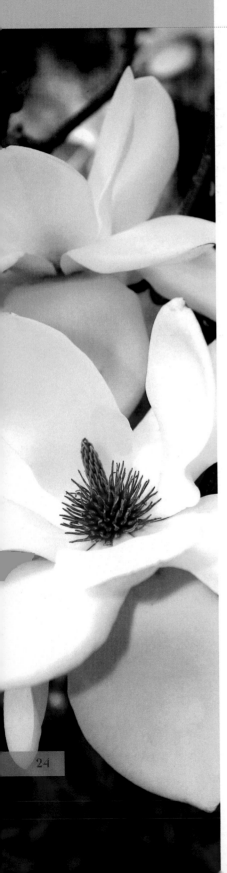

magnolia & orchid

Magnolia flowers grow on beautiful trees native to Asia and the Americas. The flowers have a large, cuplike shape with an intoxicating fragrance. The trees can grow up to 100 feet tall, producing immense blossoms ranging in color from white to purple.

The magnolia tree is a prehistoric plant. Fossilized specimens of magnolias have been found dating back almost twenty million years. This plant is said to have been on the Earth before bees. The plant developed large, thick flowers to encourage pollination by beetles. Through genetic evolution, the petals of the magnolia flowers became extremely tough to avoid damage from the large, pollinating beetles.

Traditional Chinese medicine practitioners have been using magnolia flowers, buds, and bark for centuries. Magnolia flowers are an important herb used to treat nasal congestion and sinus infections. The tree bark is used in many herbal formulas for treating acute and chronic sinus infections. The bark has been shown to have natural antibiotic properties that target strep and staph bacteria, which produce strep throat, bacterial bronchitis, and the common cold.

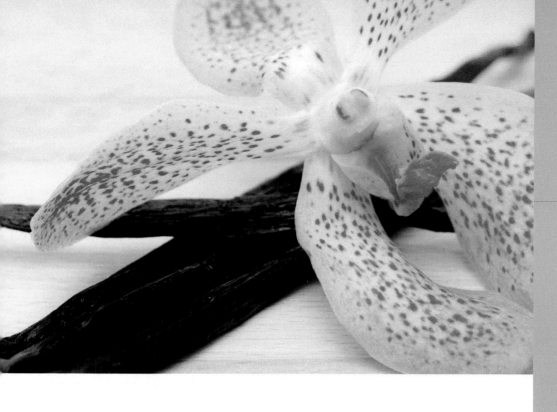

Orchids have an ancient origin and are a prehistoric plant. Some species of orchids have fossilized specimens dating back almost a million years. Orchids are part of a large family of flowers with over 20,000 different varieties. The number of orchid species is more than twice the number of bird species, and four times the number of mammal species.

Vanilla flavoring is made from the fruit of the vanilla orchid. Each pod contains thousands of tiny seeds. The pods are processed to create the vanilla extract that is used in flavoring of pastries and ice cream. Pure vanilla extract can be very expensive as these trees are mainly farmed on large plantations in Africa and Latin America.

The vanilla plant is the only orchid widely used for industrial purposes in the food and cosmetic industry. In Chinese medicine, many orchid species are used in combination with other herbs to support immune response.

Fossils of orchids have been found dating back a million years. Orchids have an ancient origin, perhaps coexisting alongside dinosaurs.

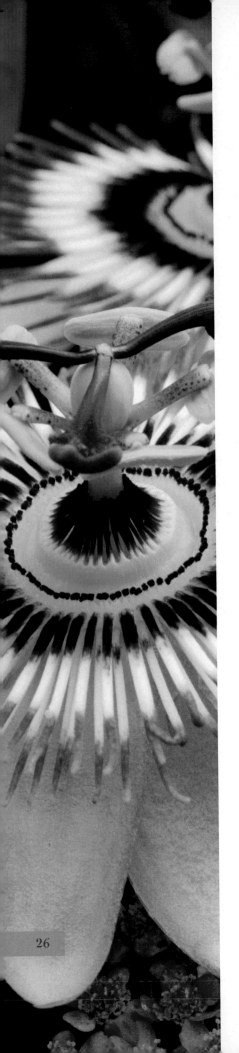

passionflower & peony

Passionflower is a beautiful vine with a very exotic-looking flower. The flowers come in a variety of colors, varying from white to orange to purple. The leaves and roots have a long history as herbal medicines in many cultures.

Passionflower is used as a natural medicine for the treatment of symptoms of anxiety and insomnia. Because of the complicated biological makeup of this plant, it has many different medicinal uses. The roots and leaves have phytochemicals that can naturally elevate serotonin. Serotonin is a neurotransmitter found in the brain that works to stabilize and elevate mood and help to regulate sleep. Another natural chemical found in this plant is *malito*, which has a strong calming effect on the nervous system.

Concentrated passionflower extract can be found at your local health food store in pill form and in tinctures. Follow the recommended dosages. Try this natural remedy at night after a stressful day to help promote a calming effect and to produce a good night's sleep.

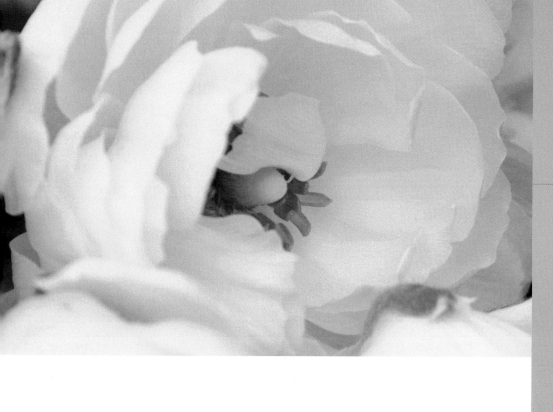

Peony is one of the most important flowers seen in Asian art. It is a classical Asian flower motif that is used on ceramics, paintings, and textiles. This flower grows on large bushes and is native to Asia, Europe, and North America. The flowers are very fragrant and can range in colors from white to yellow to red.

The peony plant has many medicinal properties. The most common reason peony is used in Chinese herbal medicine is to treat women's hormonal imbalances. Chinese herbal formulas using peony flower help to relieve menstrual cramps and reduce many symptoms of PMS. It is used with other herbs to increase ovulation and enhance fertility. Peony is one of the traditional herbs that can be used throughout a pregnancy to enrich the blood and nourish the fetus.

Peony flower and root of this plant are always mixed with other herbs to create formulas for specific types of symptoms and should be prescribed by a licensed health care practitioner.

Peony has many medicinal herbal properties. It is most commonly used in formulas to treat women's hormonal imbalances, help with mood stabilization, and beautify the skin.

27

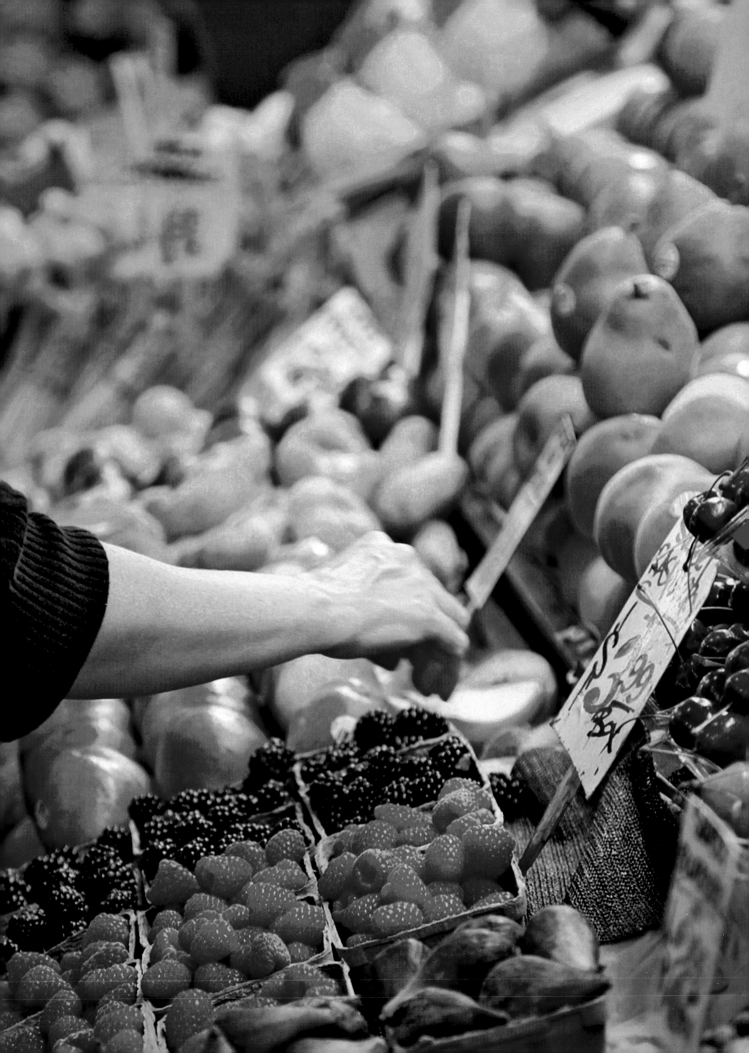

fruits:
beauty
& health

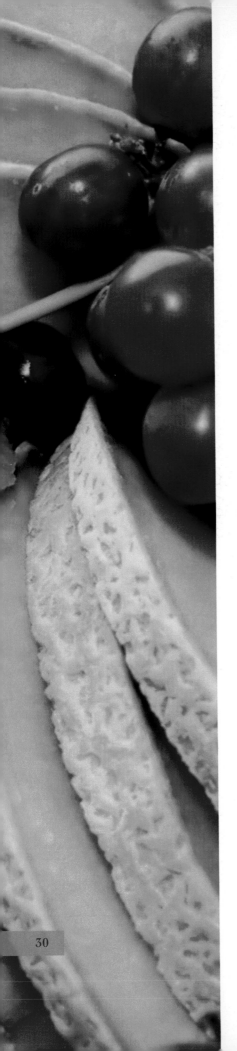

Rejuvenation & Detoxification

From the plant kingdom comes the beautiful and delicious world of exotic fruits. Because of their wonderful sweet flavors, vivid colors, and sensual textures, fruits were considered by the Greeks as the "gifts of the gods." Fruits are rich in water-soluble vitamins, enzymes, and antioxidants, and some are even high in essential fatty acids and proteins.

All fruits and most vegetables contain water-soluble vitamins that the body needs daily. Fruits also contain high levels of fiber and antioxidants that are necessary for maintaining healthy colon function and that also help to detoxify the blood.

Some of the important phytochemicals found in fruits are antioxidants. Their main job is to clean free radicals from the blood. Free radicals have been shown to cause damage to all tissues of the body. Papaya and pineapple are packed with natural digestive enzymes and help with the digestion of all foods. Coconuts, avocados, and açaí berries are high in essential fatty acids. These "good-guy" essential fats make all hormones in the body. Hormones are necessary to help regulate sleep, fertility, menstrual cycles, libido, and brain chemistry.

Choose substituting fruit for deserts over high-calorie processed sweets. Most fresh fruits will not significantly raise blood sugar levels and can also help to satisfy a sweet tooth.

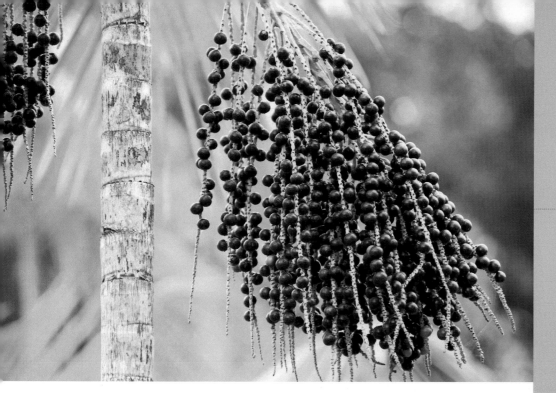

Açaí berries (pronounced "ah-sai") come from a palm tree that grows mainly in the swamps and floodplains of Brazil. These palms grow to almost 100 feet tall. The açaí berries have been used by tribes in the Amazon jungle for thousands of years as a staple food. Many parts of the tree and fruit are used for food and medicine. This fruit is a major part of the diet for many of the tribes in the Amazon today.

The berry looks like a grape and is rich in carbohydrates, vitamins, minerals, proteins, and essential fatty acids. This fruit also contains protein and natural oils, which gives it a similar nutritional value to that of coconuts, avocados, and olive oil. Essential fatty acids and antioxidants are some of the most vital nutrients for the body. Antioxidants help remove cancer-causing free radicals, and essential fatty acids make all hormones.

Açaí berries are sold at most health food stores as frozen pulp, juice, and dried powder. It is great added to smoothies, shakes, and protein drinks.

The extremely high antioxidant properties of açaí berries come from anthocyanins. These substances create the purple rich color and medicinal properties in fruits such as grapes, plums, and berries.

avocado & bananas

The essential fatty acids found in avocados, fruits, seeds, nuts, beans, and vegetables help to regulate brain function, mood, memory, and sleep. They also play a key role in the production of all hormones.

Avocado is considered one of the most nutritious fruits in the world due to its low sugar content, high protein, and rich in "good-guy" essential fatty acids. These essential fatty acids are important for heart and brain health.

In recent years, people have avoided eating avocados because of their high oil, fat, and calorie content, yet these fats and oils are, in fact, "the good-guy fats." The body cannot live without these oils, which is why they are called "essential." The essential fatty acids found in avocado help to regulate brain function, mood, memory, and sleep, and they also help with all hormone production in the body. Hormones are important for the regulation of menstrual cycles, energy production, and all adrenal hormones.

Avocado and Cilantro Butter

Avocado and cilantro blended together make a butter that is delicious served on meat, fish, and chicken. In a blender or food processor, add 3 ripe avocados, 1 bunch of cilantro (the leafy part only), 1/2 cup of avocado oil, the juice of 2 lemons, 1/2 teaspoon of salt, and 1 teaspoon of fresh cracked black pepper.

Blend for about 1 minute. The butter will be thick, creamy, and rich. It will keep for about 1 week in the refrigerator. Serve as a thick dollop on grilled lamb, fish, and chicken.

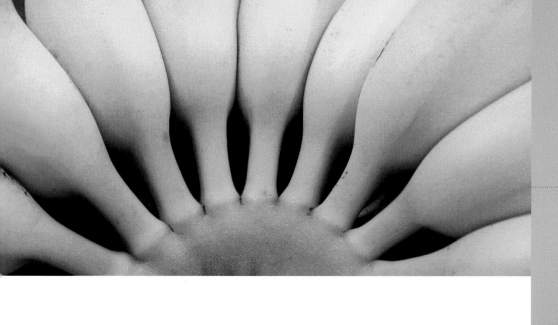

Bananas are native to Southeast Asia. Recent archaeological evidence suggests banana cultivation dates back to 8,000 BC.

Bananas come in a variety of sizes and colors including yellow, purple, and red. They are grown in over 100 different countries, and are cultivated mainly for their fruit. They are also used in making banana wine and liqueurs.

Bananas are a rich source of potassium. A single banana has more than 400 mg. of potassium. This trace mineral is important for the nervous system to function properly and helps stabilize heart rhythms and drop blood pressure. Bananas have the highest fiber content of any fruit. A study published in the *Archives of Internal Medicine* showed fruits and vegetables, high in fiber content, can help prevent cardiovascular disease.

Bananas are called "the happy fruit" as they contain tryptophan, an amino acid that converts to serotonin. When serotonin levels are high, we feel happy. Try a banana with hot milk and honey for a good night's sleep. Milk and bananas are both high in tryptophan. Milk is high in calcium, which helps to calm the nervous system. Together they have two important natural chemicals that can help you sleep, naturally.

Bananas contain an important trace mineral, potassium, which helps to stabilize and regulate heart rhythms. They are also known as the "happy fruit," as they contain amino acids that manufacture serotonin, a natural mood enhancer.

Berries and cherries contain an impressive amount of phytochemicals that reduce inflammation. They also contain high levels of vitamin C and antioxidants that can help reduce free radical damage.

Berries and cherries are some of the few fruits native to forests of North America. The dark purple juices extracted from berries were used by the Native Americans to make natural plant dyes. Dried berries were crushed into powders and rubbed onto meat for flavoring and tenderizing. In Europe, strawberries were used in many herbal medicines. Berry leaves were combined with other herbs and used to treat stomach problems.

Phytochemicals found in these fruits have a very powerful effect on lowering levels of inflammatory markers in the blood. C-reactive protein (CRP) shows how much inflammation there is in the bloodstream at the time of the testing. Chronic inflammation in the body is now considered the first stage of heart disease and cancer. Research studies have shown that high cholesterol and high blood pressure can be significantly lowered by eating diets high in fiber.

All berries and cherries are very low in natural sugar and calories. They are high in vitamins, antioxidants, and trace minerals. Berries and cherries added to plain yogurt and natural sweetener become a satisfying, healthy alternative to ice cream. They are also delicious added to smoothies and protein drinks.

berries, cherries, & coconut

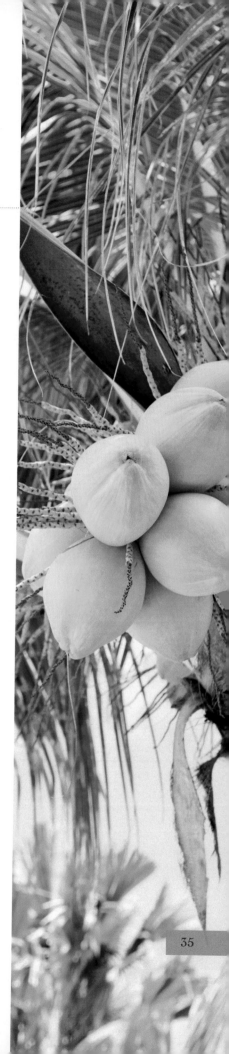

Coconut provides a nutritious source of meat, juice, and oil. For many people living in tropical countries, coconut is and has been a staple food for thousands of years. Fresh coconut meat is delicious and the nutritious coconut water can be used to make drinks and shakes. Coconut water is the clear, sweet liquid inside the coconut. It contains many vitamins, minerals, electrolytes, enzymes, and proteins. Coconut water is so close to the same chemical structure of blood plasma that it was used in hospitals during World War II as a replacement for saline IV drips.

Coconut is classified as a "complete food." That means it has proteins, vitamins, minerals, essential fatty acids, and electrolytes. The coconut palm is so highly valued by cultures in the South Pacific, both as a source of food and as a medicinal plant, that it was called "the tree of life."

Now many supermarkets carry fresh cut coconut. It is slightly sweet with a crispy, dense texture similar to a carrot. It can be eaten as a healthy, nutritious, high-protein snack. Fresh coconut water is a modern, healthy electrolyte replacement high in nutrition. Try using coconut water when making your next shake or smoothie.

Kiwi fruit has the highest concentration of magnesium of any fruit. Magnesium is a trace mineral proven to play an important role in cardiovascular health.

Kiwi is a funny-looking, fuzzy, brown fruit that grows on vines. Like grapes, the vines of the kiwi must grow and mature for several years before they will bear fruit. The vines grow rapidly, but can take anywhere from two to five years before they bear fruit. Kiwi is native to Eastern China and is now cultivated all over the world.

Kiwi has the highest concentration of magnesium of any fruit. Magnesium is a trace mineral proven to play an important role in cardiovascular health. Kiwi also contains more potassium than bananas and oranges. They are abundant in other nutrients, including folic acid, copper, pantothenic acid, calcium, iron, and vitamin B6.

Kiwi is also rich in a phytochemical called lutein. Lutein is shown to protect the eyes from developing age-related macular degeneration and cataracts.

Spicy Kiwi Salsa

Chop 4 kiwis, 1 orange, 1/2 cup of fresh pineapple, a dash of red chili flakes, 5 tablespoons of finely chopped cilantro, and 1/4 cup of finely chopped red onion, then combine. This salsa is a bright, fresh accompaniment for chicken and fish.

kiwi & papaya

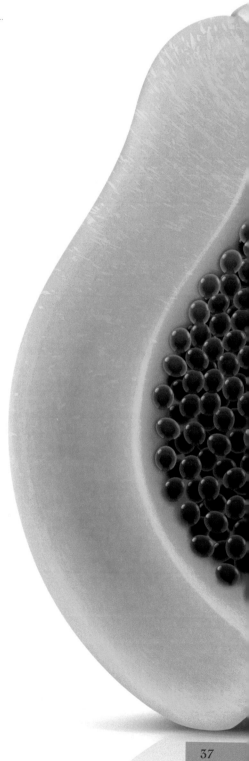

Papaya is a fruit that grows on trees in tropical climates. It is traditionally served with fresh-squeezed lime. The fruit, leaves, and seeds of this plant are used in many countries for medicinal and culinary purposes. The fruit itself is rich in an enzyme called papain. Papain is a digestive enzyme that helps with the digestion of foods, especially meat proteins.

In the South Pacific Islands, papaya and pineapple are both used as marinades and used in the preparation of many meats and fish. Green papayas, those that are not ripe, are made into salads, curries, and soups. The black seeds found inside this fruit are edible and have a sharp, spicy taste and are used like pepper. In Asia, the young leaves of papaya trees are steamed and eaten like spinach.

As we age, we naturally produce fewer digestive enzymes. These enzymes are made by the body and are signaled to enter the stomach and small intestine to help with the different phases of metabolism of food. When these enzymes are deficient, they can cause heartburn, acid reflux, constipation, gas, and bloating. Using fresh and dried papaya and papain may be a simple solution for common digestive problems. Dried papaya in pill form can be found at any health food store or vitamin shop. Try taking two tablets with every meal, and within a week, if you are enzyme deficient, symptoms such as indigestion, gas, and bloating may be greatly reduced.

Pineapple is full of vitamins, minerals, healthy fiber, and digestive enzymes. Bromelain, a natural pineapple enzyme, can be taken in a concentrated dose to help with digestive problems such as gas, bloating, and indigestion.

Pineapple is a plant native to South America, named for its resemblance to a pinecone. Christopher Columbus was credited with discovering the pineapple on the island of Guadeloupe in 1493, and took this fruit back to Europe. He called it *piña de Indes,* meaning "pinecone fruit of the Indians."

Pineapple has many vitamins, minerals, fiber, and enzymes. Enzymes are particularly good for helping with the breakdown and digestion of all food, especially heavy meat proteins. One of the most important enzymes found in pineapple is bromelain, a proteolytic enzyme or protease.

Bromelain is used in high doses before and after surgery to stop the inflammation associated with swelling caused by surgery. Ask your health care provider if this supplement could be helpful before surgery. To use bromelain for digestive problems, take 500 mg. three times a day with meals.

pineapple & watermelon

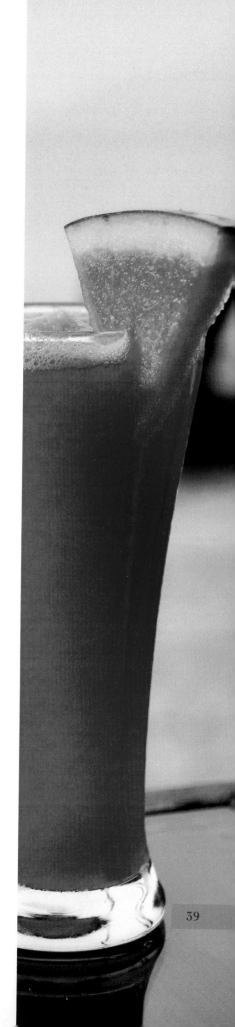

Watermelon grows in more than 1,200 varieties. It ranges in size from less than a pound, to more than two hundred pounds, and with the inside fruit varying in color from red, orange, and yellow to white. All parts of the watermelon, including the fruit, rind, and seeds, are used for their medicinal properties. They are extremely rich in iron content, as high as spinach.

All red fruits and vegetables have high concentrations of lycopene, an antioxidant and beta-carotene. All antioxidants from fruits and vegetables neutralize the harmful effects of free radicals in the human body. Free radicals cause a level of toxicity and aging to cells. In Asia and the Middle East, watermelon seeds are dried, roasted, and eaten as a snack, much like pumpkin seeds. In Africa, watermelon seeds are ground and added into soups. The seeds are very nutritious and high in proteins, fats, iron, and trace minerals.

Watermelon Lime Smoothie

Fill a blender half full with cut-up watermelon. Add a few ice cubes, the juice of 2 limes, a little natural sweetener, add water to the top, and blend for 30 seconds. This delicious, easy-to-make, healthy drink is very refreshing and nutritious. Watermelon juice is a famous drink served all over Latin America, called *aqua fresca*.

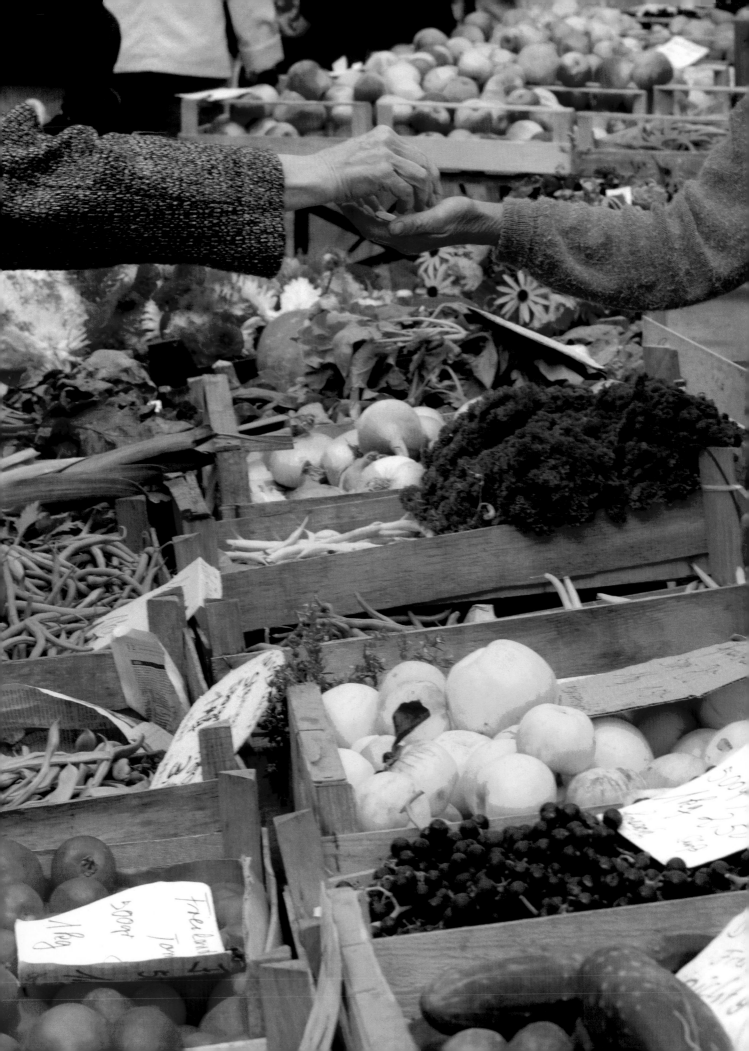

vegetables: revitalization & longevity

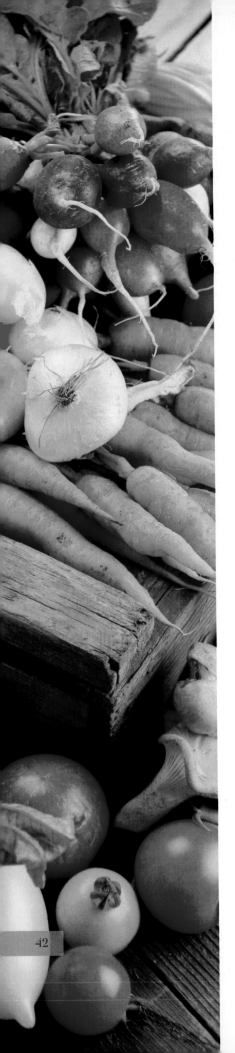

Optimum Health

Vegetables and fruits play a vital role in our health. They provide the body with the necessary vitamins, minerals, fiber, essential fatty acids, and antioxidants. These nutrients are necessary to create cellular rejuvenation.

Over the past 30 years, researchers have developed a solid base of scientific evidence to back up what generations of our mothers and grandmothers were always saying, "eat your vegetables" but nobody knew why. *The China Study,* written by T. Colin Campbell, Ph.D., and Thomas Campbell, M.D., and a Harvard-based Nurse's Health Study are two of the most comprehensive studies done on the effects of diet and health. Both of these studies had the same conclusions: The higher the daily intake of fruits and vegetables, the lower the chances of developing cardiovascular disease, cancer, and other chronic degenerative diseases.

The average American gets a total of about three servings of fruits and vegetables a day. The latest dietary guidelines call for at least five servings. An easy way to think about how to eat for optimum health is that 70% to 80% of the daily diet should be fruits and vegetables. Variety is important, as no single fruit or vegetable can provide all the vitamins, minerals, and important nutrients the body needs. Try eating lots of brightly colored fruits and vegetables to take an important step to creating a state of health and rejuvenation for your body.

Artichoke is a member of the thistle family and is native to Europe and North Africa. It was first cultivated by the Romans and Greeks and is now grown worldwide. The leaves and the "heart" of this plant are considered a delicacy in many cultures.

Artichokes are used in Chinese medicine to improve liver function. The leaves are used medicinally to increase liver bile production and to decrease lipid levels. Taking artichoke leaf extract and making diet changes can be helpful in preventing and reducing high cholesterol. Some studies show that artichoke leaf extract can help reduce elevated liver enzymes. Artichoke extract is also used to clear toxins and free radicals, known precursors to many types of illnesses.

Grilled Artichokes

Artichokes are delicious grilled. Cut artichokes in half, brush with olive oil, and sprinkle with salt and pepper. Place the artichoke halves cut-side-down on the grill. Cover and grill for 5 to 10 minutes. To serve: squeeze on fresh lemon and serve with aioli, mayonnaise, or melted butter.

The Romans and Greeks considered the artichoke to be a delicacy and an aphrodisiac. Because of their reputed potent aphrodisiac properties, only men were allowed to eat them.

43

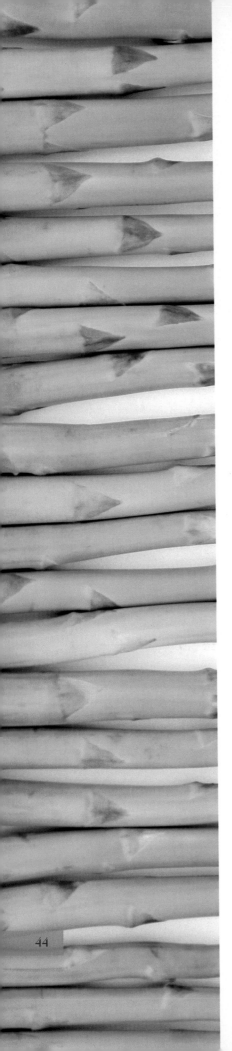

asparagus & beets

Asparagus is a vegetable native to the western coasts of Spain and Portugal. It has been considered a delicacy since ancient times. This vegetable also has a long history as a botanical medicine. In Chinese and Ayurvedic medicine, asparagus is a medicinal food used to clear out toxins stored in the liver and help regulate cholesterol. Early writings show this plant was cultivated by the Egyptians and was also a popular summer vegetable eaten by the Greeks and Romans.

Asparagus is high in many antioxidants known to help reduce chronic inflammation in the body. Inflammation is a known precursor for many illnesses such as arthritis, diabetes, and heart disease. An important antioxidant in asparagus is called saponins. This natural plant chemical is being studied for its anti-cancer properties. Another important antioxidant in asparagus is glutathione. Glutathione is one of the best-studied antioxidants and is known to support immune response by helping the production of fighter cells.

Grilled Asparagus

Asparagus is easy to make and cooks in a few minutes. It makes a delicious Chinese style stir-fry with beef, garlic, ginger, onions, and soy sauce. Grilled asparagus takes just a few minutes on the BBQ. Brush with extra virgin olive oil, fresh grated lemon zest, sea salt, and pepper. Grill for a few minutes per side and finish with a squeeze of fresh lemon.

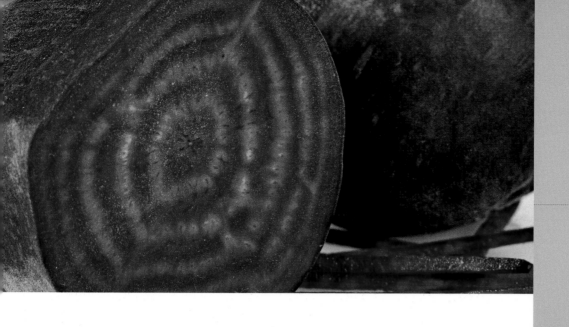

Beets contain many important vitamins and minerals, including iron and copper. The high iron content of beets helps to supply fresh oxygen to the blood. Copper is another trace mineral in beets that helps iron become more available to the cells. Because beets are so high in easily absorbable iron, they are a safe and natural remedy for some types of anemia.

Traditionally beets were only used for their medicinal properties and then became a popular culinary vegetable in the 1800s when French chefs recognized their delicious flavor. Today most garden-variety beets are deep ruby red in color, but yellow, white, and even candy-striped beets are available in specialty markets.

Roasted Beet & Arugula Salad

Use 8 whole beets, wash and peel. Place beets in a roasting pan, add 4 tablespoons olive oil, 4 tablespoons of fresh chopped rosemary, 3 cloves of fresh chopped garlic, 1/2 teaspoon salt, and 1 teaspoon of fresh cracked black pepper. Roast in the oven for 45 minutes at 350° or until beets are tender. Cut into slices. Dress arugula with olive oil, salt, pepper, and vinegar to taste. Slice warm beets into thin wedges, place on top of the cold arugula salad and sprinkle with goat cheese. Serve warm.

Well-known doctors of ancient Greece like Hippocrates, Galen, and Paracelsus used beet juice to cure fevers, anemia, and digestive problems. Beet juice is rich in easily absorbable organic iron and can be helpful for anemia.

Cruciferous vegetables contain phytochemicals called indoles. This natural plant chemical is being studied for its anticancer properties.

Cabbage, kale, brussels sprouts, broccoli, cauliflower, and collards are all members of a family of vegetables containing very specific medicinal properties that have been used for food and medicine for centuries. These vegetables are native to Asia and are thought to have been brought to Europe around 600 BC.

The phytochemicals in cruciferous vegetables are currently being studied for their anticancer enzymes. In addition, these vegetables are rich in many antioxidants that have anti-inflammatory properties. Oxidative stress and chronic inflammation in the body create a risk factor for all degenerative diseases, such as high blood pressure, high cholesterol, and the development of cancer.

The delicate flavor and crispy texture of Napa cabbage is great added to other salad greens. Baby bok choy makes a delicious cooked vegetable sautéed with garlic, ginger, onions, and soy sauce. The red color of red cabbage reflects its high concentration of antioxidants, and this variety is delicious made into a healthy, simple coleslaw combined with green apple, cilantro, green onion, olive oil, vinegar, salt, and pepper.

cabbage & celery

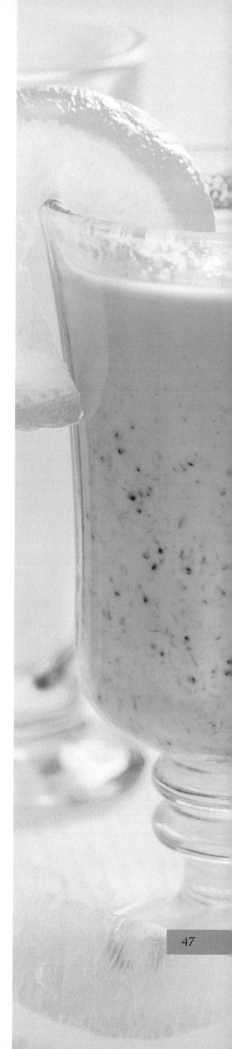

Celery can be thought of as a medicinal vegetable because it is very alkalizing to the blood. The alkalinity of the blood is like body temperature, needing to stay within a particular range. When the blood pH becomes too acidic, tissue inflammation can occur. Celery is also an excellent source of B vitamins, potassium, folic acid, calcium, magnesium, iron, phosphorus, sodium, and amino acids.

Hippocrates, the famous Greek physician, considered the "Father of Medicine," prescribed celery juice to patients suffering from nervous tension and symptoms of high blood pressure. Chinese medicine has long recognized celery to reduce high blood pressure and only recently has it been studied for its medicinal properties. The University of Chicago Medical Center studied celery's effects on blood pressure. The active plant compound, phthalides, found in celery helps to dilate blood vessels, which, in turn, reduces blood pressure. Phthalides also have been shown to reduce elevated stress hormones.

Healthy Green Drink

To make a delicious green drink using celery, wash and cut up 2 green apples, 2 carrots, 4 stalks of celery, 2 cucumbers, and 3 slices of fresh ginger. Put everything through a juicer and serve. This juice keeps well in the refrigerator for a few days.

kale & olives

Kale is rich in alphalinoleic acid, an omega-3 fatty acid that is essential for healthy brain function. Omega-3's have been shown to reduce the risk of type-2 diabetes.

Kale, like broccoli, cauliflower, and collards, is descendent from wild cabbage, a plant thought to have originated in Asia Minor.

Like most cruciferous vegetables, kale has been studied for its natural plant compounds that inhibit the growth of some types of cancer cells. Some of the most important antioxidant and anticancer compounds found in kale are called glucosinolates. Glucosinolates are a class of organic compounds found in high levels in the whole family of cruciferous vegetables. Scientists are currently interested in the potential of this plant chemical to help in the prevention of cancer.

Kale has more vitamin A than any other leafy green. One cup of chopped kale contains 133% of the recommended daily dose of vitamin A. It's also an excellent source of vitamin C.

Kale Chips

Preheat the oven to 275°. Wash and thoroughly dry 1 bunch of kale. Remove the spine of the kale leaves and cut into 1 inch pieces. Lay the chopped kale on a baking sheet and drizzle with 2 tablespoons olive oil and sea salt to taste. Bake until crisp, turning the leaves halfway through—total cooking time is about 20 minutes. Serve as a healthy salty snack that makes a great replacement for high-calorie chips.

Olive trees are native to the Mediterranean and are a favorite food in this region. There are many types of olives, ranging in color from green to black. At health food markets you can taste numerous different varieties. Some olive trees live to be over 200 years old. Olives and olive oils have been used for food, medicine, and even in soaps and skin care products.

Some of the basics of the Mediterranean diet are olives, olive oil, goat cheese, and fish. This diet has become synonymous with health, low cholesterol, and low cardiovascular risk. Olives are rich in essential fatty acids, also known as omega-3's and omega-6's. These good fats are essential for healthy brain function and hormone production.

Research shows that diets high in essential fatty acids can help lower cholesterol, lower blood pressure, and reduce the risk of cardiovascular disease.

Olive Tapenade

Olive tapenade is a rich olive spread popular in the Mediterranean. It's easy to make with just a few simple ingredients. Combine 30 pitted kalamata olives,1 tablespoon capers, 1 teaspoon fresh lemon juice, 2 teaspoons olive oil, and 1 teaspoon of fresh cracked black pepper. Place all ingredients in a blender or food processor. Makes about 1 cup. Serve on sandwiches or crackers.

Onions contain a variety of naturally occurring plant chemicals known as organo-sulfur compounds. These compounds have been linked to lowering blood pressure and cholesterol levels.

Onions include yellow, red, and white onions, as well as scallions, chives, shallots, and pearl onions. Bulbs from the onion family have been used as a food source since the Bronze Age dating back to 5,000 BC. Archaeological evidence shows that onions were a cultivated crop in Egypt. Egyptians worshipped onions, believing the spherical shape and concentric rings symbolized eternal life.

As a culinary herb, onions are an aromatic necessity, adding flavor to all kinds of savory dishes, and they also have many health benefits. Research shows onions contain generous amounts of quercetin, which helps protect the eyes against cataracts and slows down some types of tumor growth.

Onions contain a variety of naturally occurring chemicals known as organo-sulfur compounds. These compounds have been linked to lowering blood pressure and cholesterol levels. Both garlic and onions contain a photochemical called *alliin*. This important plant chemical is currently being studied for its ability to inhibit tumor growth.

Keep onions refrigerated, and cut while very cold to avoid watery eyes while chopping. Use onions, garlic, ginger, and soy sauce to add a delicious Asian flavor to any vegetable sauté.

onions & peppers

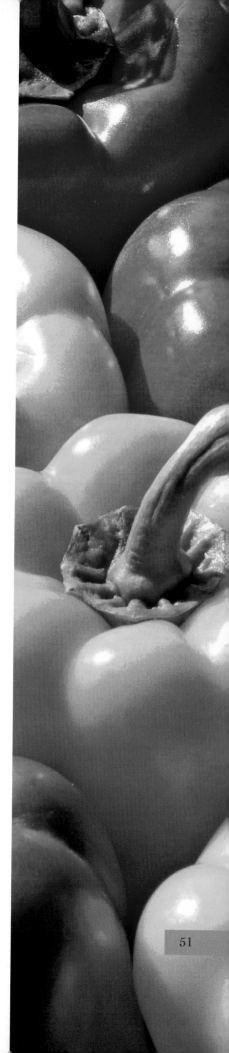

Peppers are native to Mexico and other Central American countries. Spanish and Portuguese explorers brought peppers to Europe during the 16th and 17th centuries. Bell peppers come in green, red, yellow, orange, and purplish brown and are now grown all over the world as an important commercial vegetable.

Bell peppers are chock-full of vitamin C. This vitamin is especially concentrated in the red bell peppers. Vitamin C is a potent, water-soluble antioxidant required for collagen production in the body. Collagen is the main structural protein required for maintaining the integrity of blood vessels and skin elasticity.

Pepper Chips

For a great low-calorie, high-protein snack, cut up a platter of colorful peppers. To one cup of Greek yogurt, add 1/4 cup of chives, the juice of 2 lemons, salt, and fresh ground black pepper to taste, and stir in 2 tablespoons of olive oil. The olive oil will give a delicious richness to the yogurt and provide essential fatty acids. This dip is high in protein and low in calories, and the peppers are high in vitamin C.

51

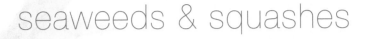

Seaweed is used extensively as food in coastal cuisines around the world and is a staple food in Asia. Seaweed is popular in Europe, especially in Ireland and Scotland where it is made into crackers. Besides being a traditional food in many countries, it has important therapeutic and medicinal benefits.

Edible seaweeds are found and harvested directly from the ocean and also cultivated as a farmed crop. It is an excellent source of many naturally occurring trace minerals, especially iodine. This mineral helps to regulate and stimulate the thyroid gland. Thyroid hormones govern metabolism, body weight, and energy. Seaweed is a food that not only can help metabolism, but is also high in natural iron, necessary for preventing iron deficiency anemia.

There are many different types of seaweed, all with slightly different tastes and textures. Japanese restaurants offer a variety of the myriad types of seaweed. Green seaweed salad has a fresh, crispy texture and a slightly salty taste. Another type of seaweed salad is called *hiziki* salad. This is a black seaweed salad made with fried tofu, ginger, soy sauce, and green onions. The most well-known seaweed is *nori*. This is the dark green seaweed that comes in thin pressed sheets and is used to wrap sushi rolls.

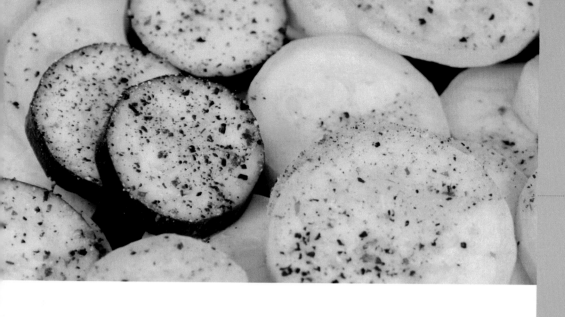

Squash was cultivated in the Americas dating back to 10,000 years ago. Summer squashes include zucchini, patty pan, and crookneck squash. Winter squashes include butternut, acorn, spaghetti, and pumpkin.

Scientific studies have shown fruits and vegetables with bright colors indicate high amounts of antioxidants. Several recent studies have shown that all types of squash contain an abundance of antioxidants and B vitamins. Squash also provides high amounts of fiber and contain a polysaccharide fiber-like pectin that helps to stabilize and regulate blood sugar levels. To keep blood sugar stable, the body requires ample amounts of B vitamins and dietary fiber, which squash contains.

Mediterranean-Style Spaghetti Squash

Spaghetti squash can make a great pasta-like dish. Carefully stab with a knife so that the steam can escape. Bake in the oven at 350° for about 1 hour or until the squash turns light brown and is slightly collapsed. Let sit for about 10 minutes to cool. Cut the squash in half and remove the seeds. Fluff up the squash inside the shell and drizzle with 2 to 3 tablespoons of olive oil, add salt and pepper to taste. Sprinkle with goat cheese and chopped, pitted kalamata olives. Finish with fresh arugula, green onions, and chopped tomatoes. Serve warm. Delicious!

Squash has been cultivated in the Americas for at least 10,000 years. In Chinese medicine, many different types of summer and winter squash are used as medicinal foods to reduce inflammation in the colon.

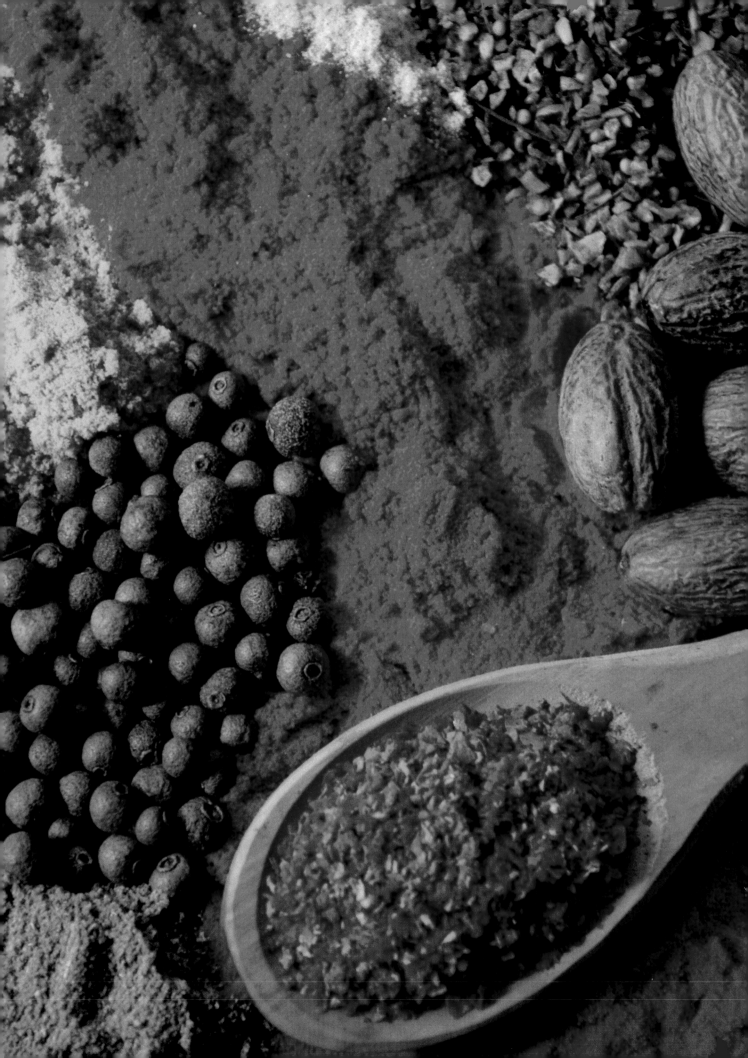

spices:
aroma
& vitality

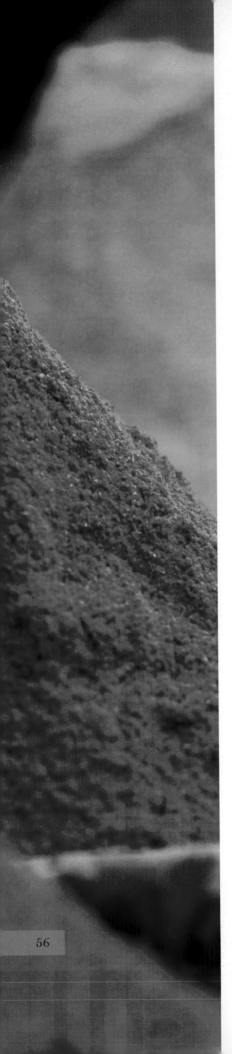

Stimulating Medicinals

Spices were some of the most important traded commodities of the ancient world. Many wars were fought and fortunes made over the spice trade. Spices add flavor to sweet or savory dishes and can make ordinary dishes exciting. Spices have a long list of health benefits. They are used topically on the skin to reduce pain and inflammation, improve cardiovascular health, stimulate immune response, and stabilize blood sugar. Many spices possess antimicrobial and natural antibiotic properties.

In Chinese and Ayurvedic medicine, spices are some of the most potent medicinal plants used alone and in combination with other botanicals. They are used fresh and dried, as well as made into liquid herbal tinctures, powders, and tablets. Spices are wonderful powerhouses of flavor and nutrients that also have many medicinal benefits.

All spices have medicinal properties. Cinnamon is known to help control blood sugar levels and aid with insulin resistance. Turmeric's key active ingredient is curcumin, used to reduce inflammation. Saffron is being studied for its promising cancer prevention benefits.

Explore new recipes and see which spices are the most interesting and exciting to your palate. Sweet spices are delicious and easy to add to smoothies, hot cereals, and baked goods. Earthy, pungent, and hot spices are great paired with stir-fry vegetable dishes, meats, fish, and poultry.

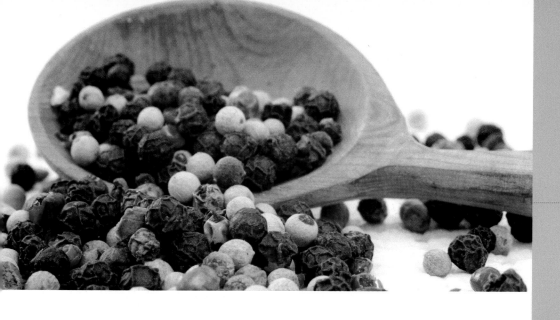

Black pepper was one of the most valuable exports in ancient times. Pepper was used as a medicinal spice, and before refrigeration, pepper was used as a preservative for poultry, meat, and fish. Consumption of pepper grew dramatically in the days of the Roman Empire and became one of the most valuable and traded spices in Europe. Pepper is still one of the world's most traded spices and is used in cuisines around the world.

One of the important medicinal properties of pepper is an alkaloid called piperine. This natural plant chemical is what gives pepper its strong, spicy, and pungent flavor. Piperine has been shown to increase hydrochloric acid in the stomach and increase enzyme production in the gastrointestinal tract, which aids in digestion. Enzymes are necessary to help with the digestion of all foods, especially proteins.

Use pepper on food to help stimulate digestion. Pepper is one of the most versatile spices as it can be used to enhance the flavor in all savory dishes, including meats, fish, and vegetables. There are many delicious types of peppercorns, such as white, red, green, and black. All have slightly different and distinct aromas and flavors. All spices are more flavorful when they are freshly ground.

Black pepper is a medicinal spice that helps stimulate digestive enzymes. Enzymes are essential in the breakdown and digestion of all food.

57

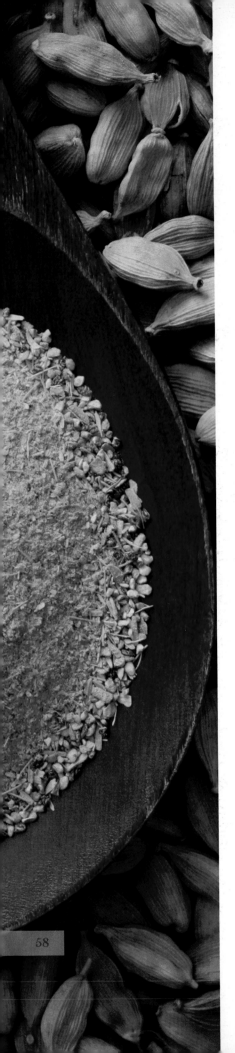

cardamom & cayenne pepper

Cardamom is native to southern India and grows throughout China and other parts of Southeast Asia. Cardamom seeds are used in many traditional herbal remedies. The pods are picked just before ripening and then sun-dried.

Cardamom is an important spice in Indian, North African, and Middle Eastern cuisines, popular in curries and savory dishes. In the Middle East, coffee is brewed with cardamom pods and served with cream and sugar. In the Scandinavian countries, this spice is used in all types of sweet pastries and bread.

Studies have also shown that some of the natural medicinal compounds in cardamom kill *H-pylori* bacteria, a common stomach bacteria that causes gastroesophageal reflux disease (GERD) and stomach ulcers.

Cardamom is used in many Chinese medicine formulas to treat symptoms such as gas, bloating, nausea, and constipation. These formulas can only be prescribed by a trained health care professional.

Cardamom Coffee

To make traditional Middle Eastern coffee, add 5 cardamom pods to 6-8 tablespoons of fresh ground coffee in a french coffee press. Add 2 cups of hot water, stir, and let set for 3 minutes to allow the flavors to combine. Add cream and natural sweetener to taste.

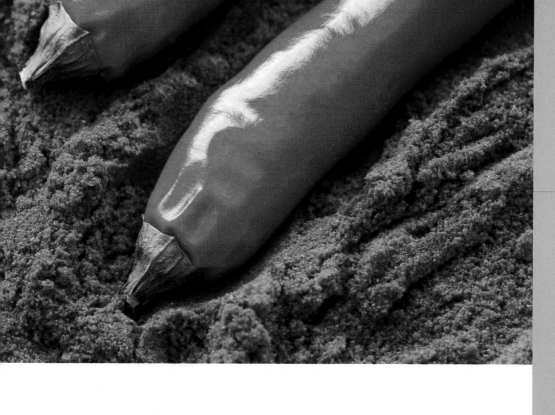

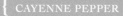

Cayenne pepper is a very small, red, hot chili pepper. After harvesting, it is dried, baked, ground, and sifted to make this potent spice. It is one of the important spices used to make many BBQ rubs, chili sauces, and hot sauces.

This red, hot chili pepper is very high in vitamins A, C, and E. Capsaicin is the natural plant alkaloid in chili peppers that gives them their heat. When this compound is applied topically to the skin it causes a warm, numbing sensation to the nerves and becomes an effective treatment for pain.

In Ayurvedic and Chinese medicine, cayenne pepper is used internally and externally to treat many different illnesses. One traditional Ayurvedic remedy for pain uses cayenne pepper and mustard seeds, which are combined into a paste and applied topically to the skin to treat arthritis.

Many over-the-counter creams and plasters, such as Zostrix and Heet, contain capsaicin. Creams containing capsaicin are used to treat pain caused from rheumatic, arthritic, and fibromyalgia conditions.

Capsaicin is the natural plant alkaloid in chili peppers, which gives them their heat. This is a common ingredient found in many over-the-counter topical pain relievers.

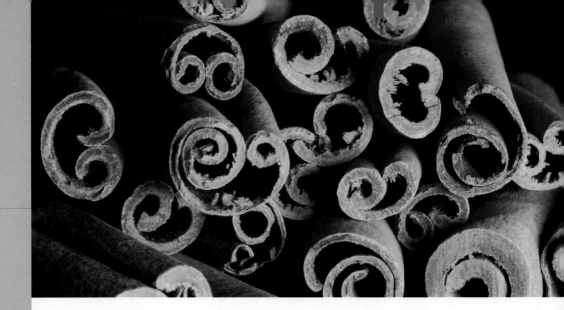

Cinnamon was so highly prized among European nations during the Middle Ages that it was regarded as a gift given to kings. This delicious sweet spice is used to help regulate blood sugar levels.

Cinnamon is found in ancient Chinese writings and used medicinally for colds, flu, and digestive issues. The ancient Egyptians used cinnamon for embalming mummies, for its pleasant scent and preservative properties.

Cinnamon is used in sweet baked goods and savory meat dishes in Indian and Middle Eastern cuisines. The Bible mentions the use of cinnamon when Moses is commanded to use sweet cinnamon and cassia in the holy anointing oils. This spice was so highly prized among the European nations during the Middle Ages that it was regarded as a gift for royalty.

In Chinese herbal medicine, cinnamon is used in combination with ginseng, ginger, and astragalus to help support immune response. Some clinical studies have shown cinnamon enhances the body's ability to use the insulin it already produces and stabilize blood sugar levels. Cinnamon used in concentrated amounts has been shown to be a simple and effective natural treatment for hypoglycemia.

Cinnamon Tea

For blood sugar stabilization, use 1/2 teaspoon of powdered cinnamon to 1 cup of hot water. Sweeten with stevia, a noncaloric natural sweetener, and drink 3 cups a day, between meals.

cinnamon & coriander

Coriander is a seed that grows into a type of parsley called cilantro, or Chinese parsley. The leaves of this plant have a very pungent, spicy taste, and it is commonly used in many Asian and Latin dishes. The seeds of the plant are dried, ground, and roasted, giving it a nutty and spicy flavor.

As a medicine, in many traditional cultures coriander seeds are made into teas and used for the treatment of the common cold and digestive symptoms. In traditional Chinese medicine, coriander is considered pungent, warming, and used in combination with other herbs to treat conditions such as stomachaches and nausea.

Just before using, put spices in a blender or in a small, clean coffee grinder and use them as freshly ground as possible. Spices are fragile and they will not have some of their exciting flavor, aroma, and potency when they have not been freshly ground.

Mediterranean Warm Spicy Lentil Salad

Add 1 teaspoon each of cumin, coriander, and black peppercorns, and grind together. Add 1/4 teaspoon of ground cardamom powder to the finished powder mixture. Mince 2 small cloves of fresh garlic and add the whole mixture to 3 cups of cooked warm lentils. Toss beans and ground spices with 5 tablespoons of extra virgin olive oil. Just before serving, add 1/4 cup of finely chopped cilantro and salt to taste. Serve warm.

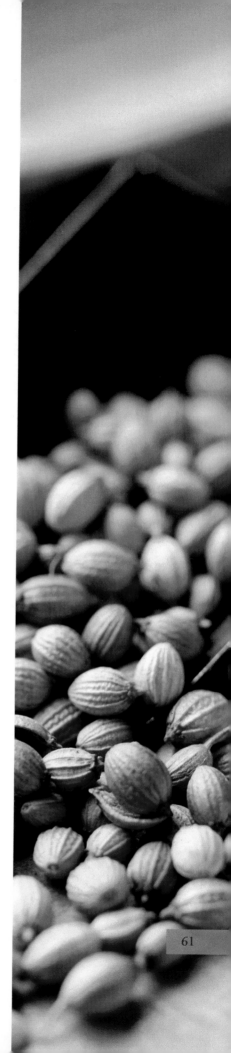

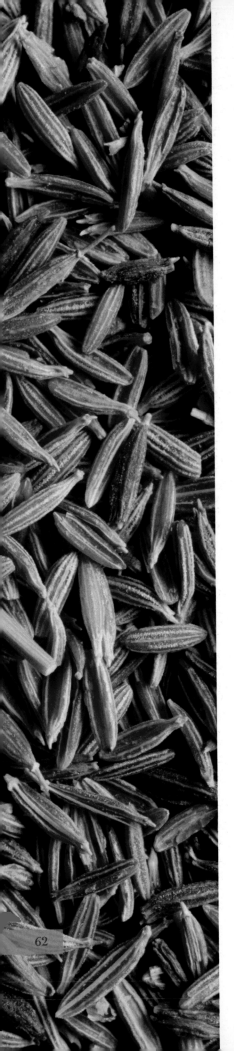

cumin & ginger

Cumin is the oblong-shaped seed of a small, flowering herb related to the parsley family. Like both dill and parsley, cumin has a strong, distinctive flavor. Cumin originated in the Mediterranean and was used as a spice and medicine by the Greeks, Romans, Egyptians, and Persians.

The Greeks used cumin much like we use pepper today. They would keep containers of ground cumin at the dinner table to sprinkle on food. This practice is still common in Middle Eastern countries. Ancient Egyptians used this spice in combination with many other spices in their mummification process.

Cumin seeds are rich in iron. Iron is an essential mineral that helps in the formation of hemoglobin. Hemoglobin in the blood is required so that oxygen can be transported into the cells. In addition, cumin helps stimulate the secretion of enzymes, which are necessary for the metabolism and breakdown of all foods.

Cumin Pepper

If you love pepper, and you want to try a new interesting spice, put 1/4 cup of cumin seeds in a small, clean coffee grinder. Blend to coarse ground. Put it in a pepper shaker and use as an exciting, pungent, peppery spice that is great on all vegetable and savory dishes.

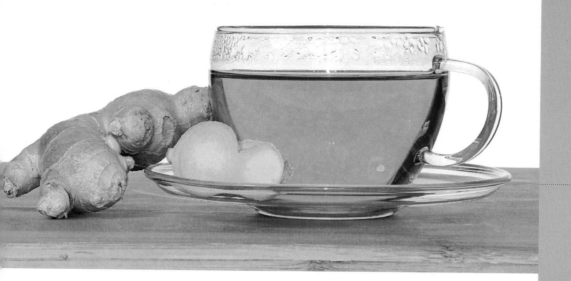

Ginger grows in tropical areas around the world in many different varieties. The root of the plant is used as a pungent spice for cooking and as a medicinal spice for digestive problems. The ancient Hawaiians used one type of the ginger flower, *awapuhi*, to make a foaming ingredient for shampoo that is still used in many commercial shampoo products today.

In most Asian cuisines, garlic, ginger, and soy sauce are some of the most basic ingredients that flavor vegetable and meat dishes. Garlic is said to be *yang* and heating, and ginger is said to be *yin* and slightly cooling. If they are paired together, they balance each other.

The active medicinal compounds in ginger are zingerone, shogaols, and gingerols. These active ingredients have been studied for their natural healing properties effective in the treatment of many digestive problems, especially nausea. Raw ginger can be used as a safe and effective natural herbal treatment by pregnant women for morning sickness.

Hot Ginger Tea

For stomach upset, peel and grate 2 heaping tablespoons of fresh ginger root. Add hot water and 1 tablespoon of honey, steep for a few minutes. Do not strain, but drink the grated ginger for a more medicinal effect.

In tropical countries ginger is a common seasoning and medicinal herb. The ancient Hawaiians used awapuhi, a specific type of ginger flower, to make shampoo. This flower is still used in many commercial shampoo products.

The state of Illinois grows 85% of the world's horseradish. It is considered the horseradish capital of the world and every year has an international horseradish festival.

Horseradish is a perennial plant related to mustard, cabbage, brussels sprouts, and other cruciferous vegetables. Horseradish root has been used in Europe and Asia as a medicinal food and in combination with other medicinal botanicals to treat sinus infections.

This whole family of cruciferous vegetables is now being studied for their anticancer properties. Horseradish root contains significant amounts of cancer-fighting compounds called glucosinolates. This natural plant chemical has been shown to increase the liver's ability to detoxify carcinogens and suppress some types of tumor cells.

Yogurt & Horseradish Sauce

Mix 1 cup of thick, low-fat Greek yogurt, 2 to 3 teaspoons of fresh grated horseradish, the juice of 2 lemons, 3 tablespoons of olive oil, 1/4 cup of water, and salt and pepper to taste. Fresh horseradish root is available in many supermarkets and is much sweeter and less pungent than the dried spice. This low-fat creamy sauce is delicious paired with roast beef, steak, chicken, pork, and beef sausages.

horseradish & mustard

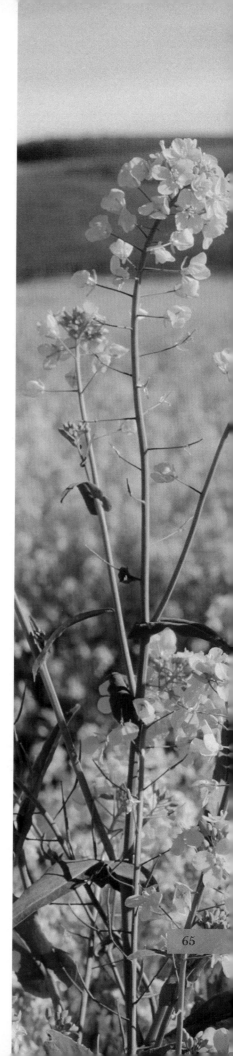

Mustard seeds are mentioned in ancient Sanskrit writings dating back almost 5,000 years. The Bible calls mustard "the greatest among the herbs," valued for its intense flavor and healing properties. Mustard seeds are used for cooking and herbal remedies, and mustard greens are a staple vegetable in many cultures. Mustard greens are an excellent source of vitamin E, vitamin C, and beta-carotene.

White and yellow mustard seeds are used extensively in the production of American mustards. Brown mustard is native to Asia and brown mustard seeds are used to make specialty mustards such as Dijon mustard.

In Chinese medicine, white mustard seeds have warming properties and interact with the lung and stomach meridians. It is used in combination with other herbs to clear dampness and phlegm from the lungs.

Sautéed Mustard Greens

In a large frying pan, add 4 tablespoons of olive oil, 1 tablespoon of ground mustard seeds, 1 large chopped white onion, and 4 cloves of chopped garlic. Stir-fry this mixture until the onions are slightly cooked. Chop 1 whole head of Chinese mustard greens into 1-inch lengths and add them to pan. Add 1/4 cup water and 2 tablespoons of soy sauce, cover, stir, and cook until the greens are tender.

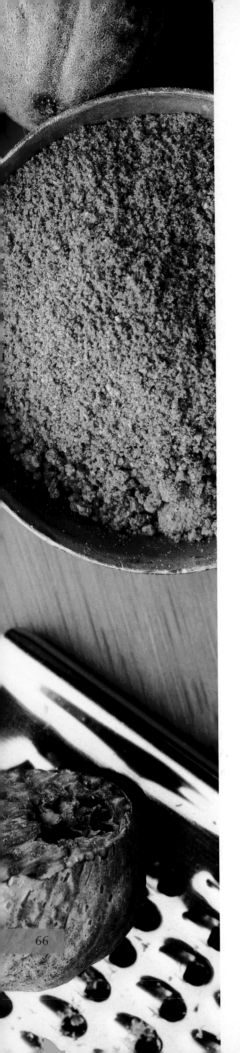

nutmeg & paprika

Nutmeg has a rich and exotic history as the spice trade became a huge business in Europe and the Middle East during the Middle Ages.

Nutmeg comes from the Banda Islands, part of the Indonesian island chain. It is a yellow, hard fruit that grows on an evergreen tree.

Nutmeg is used in Middle Eastern cuisine as a spice for savory meat and vegetable dishes. In the United States and Europe, it predominates as a sweet spice for making pumpkin pie, fruit cake, and eggnog.

Studies have shown that the compound macelignan, isolated from nutmeg, has a strong antimicrobial effect against bacterial strep infections that are common in the intestines. In Chinese medicine, it is used in combination with other herbs for the treatment of dysentery and bacterial infections caused by food poisoning. Nutmeg also helps to reduce symptoms associated with other digestive problems, such as nausea and vomiting.

As an herbal medicine, nutmeg is always used with other spices and herbs for digestive problems. Please consult a health care practitioner for these formulas.

Paprika is the powdered spice made from red bell peppers. The most common paprika is made from the sweet red pepper called tomato peppers. The powder ranges from bright red to brown and its flavor varies from sweet and mild, to pungent and hot. The hot paprika gives your taste buds a jolt. Both varieties are generally carried in most supermarkets and gourmet stores.

Many Spanish and Portuguese recipes use paprika for soups, stews, and casseroles. In India, it is used with other spices for *tandoori* chicken, which produces its beautiful red color. In Spain, paprika is used to flavor many seafood dishes. Paprika and other peppers contain capsaicin. This natural plant compound has proven effects in reducing some types of inflammation. Capsaicin is used to treat arthritis pain and joint inflammation as it has many natural anti-inflammatory properties. Many over-the-counter topical creams for the treatment of pain contain capsaicin.

Healthy Sweet Potato Fries

Cut 3 large sweet potatoes into 1/2 inch lengths and 1/2 inch widths, sprinkle lightly with paprika, 1/2 teaspoon salt, and brush with 2 tablespoons of olive oil. Bake in the oven for 20 minutes at 350°. Use paprika liberally on poultry, meat, and fish, to give a sweet and slightly spicy flavor.

Paprika is popular worldwide, but nowhere is it more popular than in Hungary, where there is a museum dedicated to this spice. Paprika was introduced to Europe from the New World by Spanish explorers.

Dried saffron can be found at many supermarkets as well as most Asian markets. Saffron is traditionally used in cooking seafood dishes such as bouillabaisse and paella.

Saffron is the yellow stigmas from the small, purple crocus flower. It is the world's most expensive spice. In order to produce one pound of dried saffron it takes approximately 75,000 flowers, or three acres of harvested flowers. Because it is so labor intensive to grow and harvest this flower, saffron is very costly and one ounce usually retails for about $40. This flower is native to Southern Europe and is now cultivated worldwide.

Saffron-based pigments have even been found in 30,000-year-old cave depictions in northwestern Iran. When Alexander the Great invaded Asia, he would use saffron in his baths to help heal battle wounds. Saffron was also traditionally used to give the golden yellow color to the robes worn by Buddhist monks.

In Chinese medicine, its main functions are to treat conditions such as high fevers and to help break up blood clots. Some studies show that saffron can inhibit the growth of some types of cancer cells.

Since heat releases saffron's flavor and beautiful color, it is best steeped in hot water before being used in cooking. Saffron is traditionally used in seafood dishes such as *bouillabaisse* and *paella* and is also delicious used in risotto and other rice dishes.

saffron & turmeric

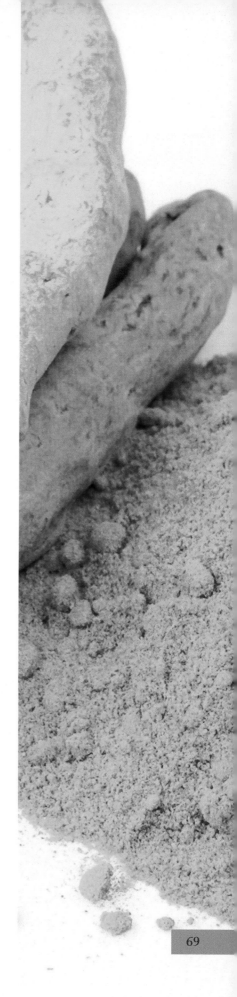

Turmeric is a member of the ginger family and native to Southeast Asia. The root of the plant is boiled, dried, and ground to make a powder. Turmeric is one of the main spices used in all Indian and Thai curry dishes.

Rich in antioxidants, turmeric has been used as an herbal medicine for thousand of years. Scientists are now studying turmeric for its anti-tumor and anti-inflammation compounds, curcuminoids, that are powerful antioxidants.

Antioxidants are important for stopping damage to cell walls caused by free radicals. Antioxidants have been studied for their capability to reverse and inhibit damage to DNA. Turmeric is used in many herbal remedies in Oriental Medicine. This herb is used to treat inflammation in all tissues in the body and is especially effective for decreasing inflammation in joints caused by arthritis.

Curry Vegetables

Turmeric can be used for adding an exciting spicy taste to all vegetable dishes. It is a delicious and simple way to brighten any stir-fry. Just add 1 tablespoon of powdered turmeric, a little water, and soy sauce at the end of cooking any vegetable dish to add an extra spicy, delicious flavor.

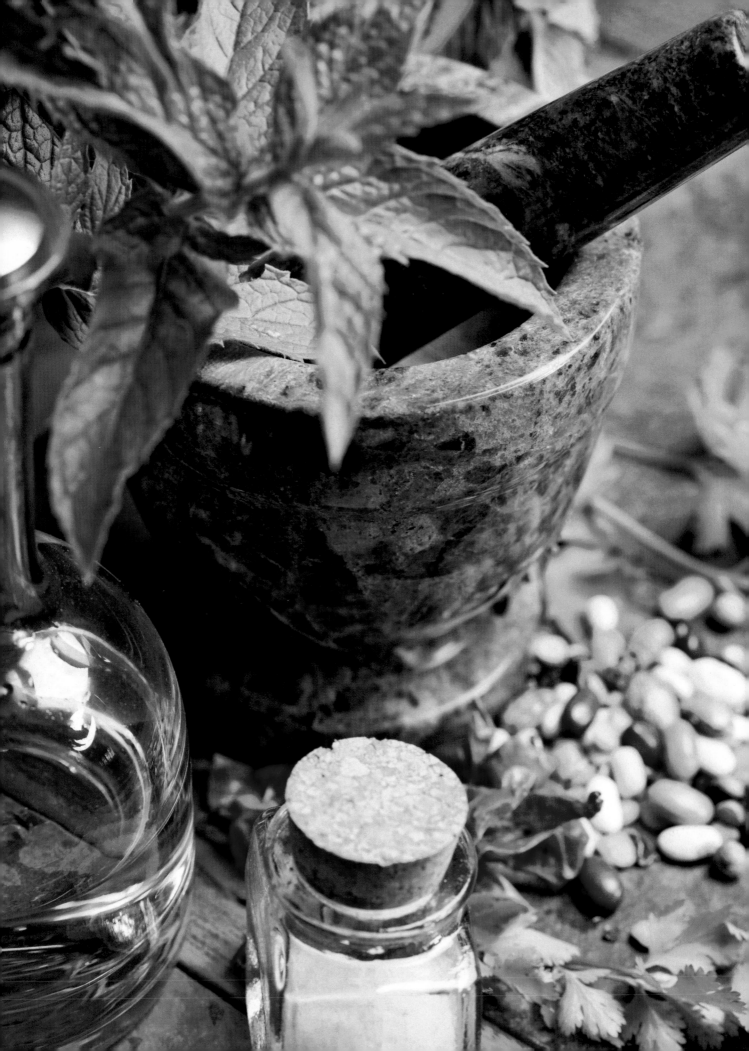

herbs: flavorful rejuvenation

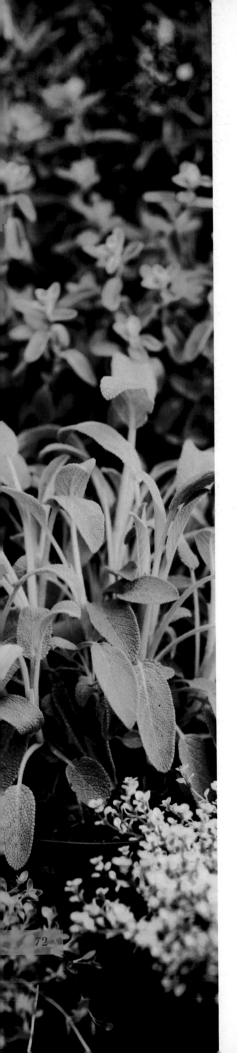

Exciting Aromatics

Herbs are full of vitamins, minerals, and antioxidants, and can add exciting aroma and flavor to any dish. All herbs are as nutritious as vegetables and have many more concentrated power-packed phytochemicals.

An easy way to start incorporating herbs into your daily diet is to buy them fresh and add a handful of fresh herbs to any type of salad. Basil, parsley, cilantro, and dill are especially good with raw vegetables, and they also add lots of flavor and color.

Herbs are a great way to add flavor to foods without adding calories or salt. There are certain classic pairings. Basil goes well with tomato and mozzarella. Dill is delicious on baked salmon and great with salad greens. Rosemary adds delightful flavor to grilled lamb, chicken, and roasted and baked vegetables.

Herbs are some of the easiest plants to grow. They grow profusely and most require very little maintenance. It is easy to make a small herb section in any garden, and they even grow well indoors by a kitchen window with natural light.

Whether you like to cook or just like to eat, an herb garden can become a source of fragrant, delicious, medicinal seasonings that will also add a lot of flavor to your favorite dishes.

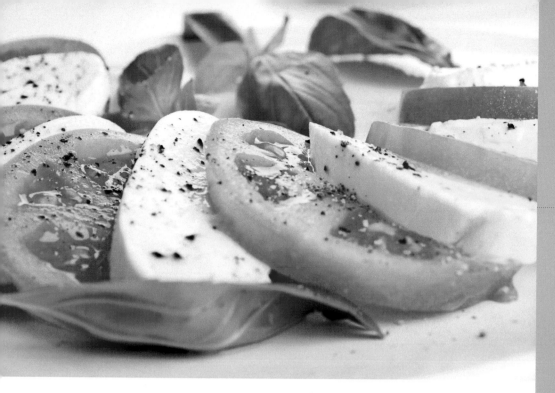

Basil is a common culinary herb known for its strong, pungent taste and very aromatic fragrance. Originally native to India and other tropical regions of Asia, basil is now used around the world in many different cuisines. Called the "king of herbs," basil comes in more than 30 varieties, with leaves ranging from bright green to deep purple. Basil can have very distinctive flavors with notes of cinnamon, lemon, and licorice.

Some early writings indicate that basil has been cultivated for more than 3,000 years. In some parts of Europe, basil was placed in the hands of the dead to ensure a safe journey into the afterlife. In India, basil was put in the mouth of the dying so that the deceased reached the afterlife.

Several scientific studies have shown the medicinal properties of basil oil has the ability to inhibit several types of common bacteria, such as staph and strep.

This herb is used in many Asian cuisines and in Italy it is used to make pesto sauce. Basil pesto is easy to make and also serves as a great sauce that can be used to add extra flavor for cooked vegetables and fish.

Concentrated basil oil is effectively used as a natural plant-based antibiotic. It has been shown to inhibit several types of bad bacteria that are common to the large and small intestines.

73

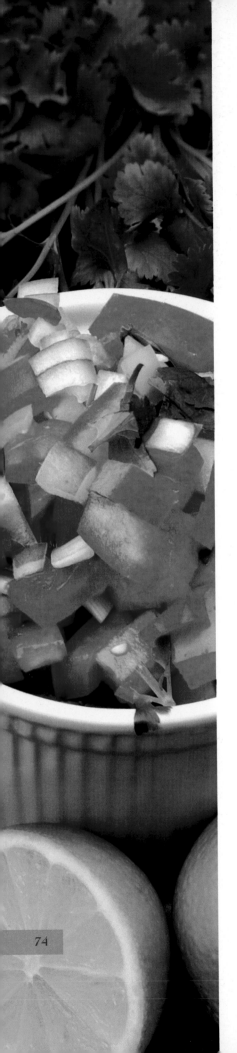

cilantro & dill

Cilantro is a type of parsley that is spicy and has a slightly bitter taste. It is also known as Chinese parsley. This plant is native to southern Europe and North Africa. Cilantro, as a culinary herb, is used primarily in Chinese, Thai, and Latin American dishes. The fresh leaves are a key ingredient in foods such as chutney, salsa, and guacamole.

Cilantro has also been used as a natural herbal remedy and was written about by the famous Greek physician Hippocrates in the *Materia Medica, 500 BC.* The natural plant chemical compounds in cilantro are currently being studied for their ability to bind and help remove heavy metals found in body tissues. The most common metals are mercury and lead. Mercury is high in metal dental fillings and fish high on the food chain, such as tuna and swordfish. Lead is common to paint, pottery, and gasoline. These metals enter the blood stream and are stored in body fat. They are known to create free radicals in the body and can cause cell degeneration and damage to DNA.

Spicy Salsa

To make a delicious fresh salsa, use 3 large fresh tomatoes finely chopped. Add 1/4 cup finely chopped red onion, 1 finely chopped serrano chile, 3/4 cup chopped fresh cilantro, 1/2 teaspoon salt, and 3 tablespoons of fresh-squeezed lime juice. Mix all ingredients together and chill for 1 hour before serving. Serve with grilled meats, fish, chips, and guacamole.

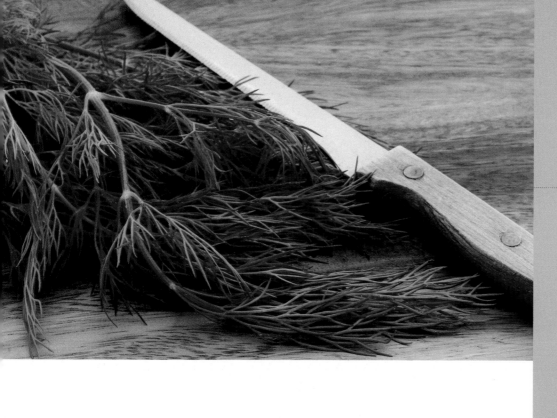

Dill is a native plant found in Russia, Africa, and the Mediterranean. It is referenced in the Bible and ancient Egyptian writings, as a culinary herb and medicinal plant. The leaves are dark green, delicate, and fern-like. The seeds are similar in taste to caraway, but have a more citrus sweet flavor.

Much like parsley, the natural plant phytochemicals in dill have been shown to neutralize some types of carcinogens in the body. Dill has also been studied for its ability to prevent bacterial overgrowth. Dill, garlic, and other common culinary herbs help to reduce many types of bacteria that are common to the large and small intestines. The seeds are used in Chinese herbal formulas for stomachache and a variety of digestive symptoms.

Dill is a favorite herb used to accent the flavor of poached salmon. Fresh dill can be found in most grocery stores and is a delicious way to add bright flavor, extra color, and texture to all types of salads and fish dishes.

Dill contains phytochemicals that have been shown to neutralize some carcinogens in the body. Fresh dill can add a bright flavor and interesting texture to all types of salads.

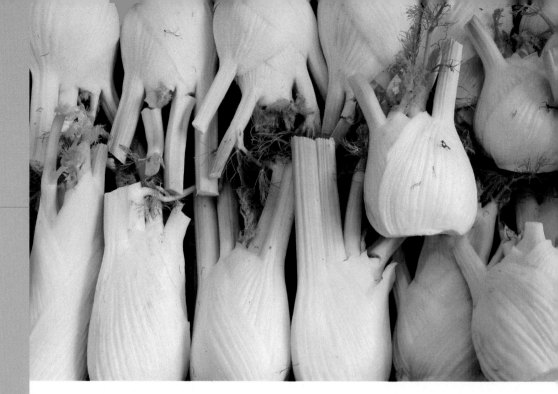

Ancient Roman texts mention the value of this plant for its aromatic seeds and medicinal properties. Fresh fennel is a delicious, spicy, aromatic, leafy green vegetable that can add a new dimension of flavor to any salad.

Fennel is a beautiful vegetable/herb that looks like celery. It has a rich spicy flavor and a texture similar to cabbage. It is delicious used as a raw salad green and in the Mediterranean is a popular cooked vegetable. The stalks and bulb can be sautéed, stewed, braised, and grilled. Fennel seed is a common ingredient in Italian sausages, meatballs, and rye breads.

Fennel is an excellent source of vitamin C, one of the body's primary water-soluble antioxidants able to neutralize free radicals. Free radicals cause cell damage that can result in inflammation in all tissues in the body. Inflammation is shown to be a precursor of many types of diseases.

Baked Fennel with Parmesan

Combine 4 tablespoons olive oil, 4 cloves of finely chopped garlic, 4 fennel bulbs cut horizontally into 1 inch thick slices, 1/2 teaspoon of salt, and 1 tablespoon of freshly ground black pepper. Mix all ingredients together and sprinkle with 1/2 cup shredded Parmesan cheese. Cover and bake for 45 minutes at 375°. Serve warm.

fennel & garlic

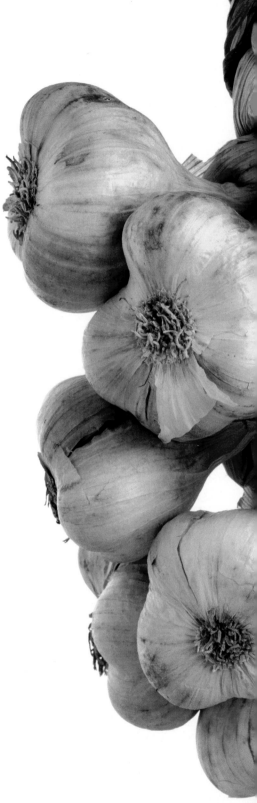

Garlic is related to the onion family. The garlic plant's bulb is divided into numerous fleshy sections called cloves. The cloves are used both raw and cooked for medicinal purposes. Throughout history garlic has been used both as a culinary herb and as a natural medicine.

The myth that garlic wards off evil spirits comes from the ancient Greeks. Garlic was said to be placed outside as a food for Hecate, the Greek goddess of the wilderness and childbirth. Garlic was made into wreaths and hung in doorways to scare away evil spirits from entering a house.

In Russia and Japan, garlic has been studied for its particular medicinal properties. Studies have shown that garlic is effective in the inhibition of strep and staph bacteria.

Garlic can be used in preparing any kind of savory dishes, from meats and seafood, to grains, pasta, and vegetables. It adds an extremely potent aroma and exceptional flavor. Garlic pairs well with many other spices and herbs and is a staple spice used in many Asian and Italian dishes.

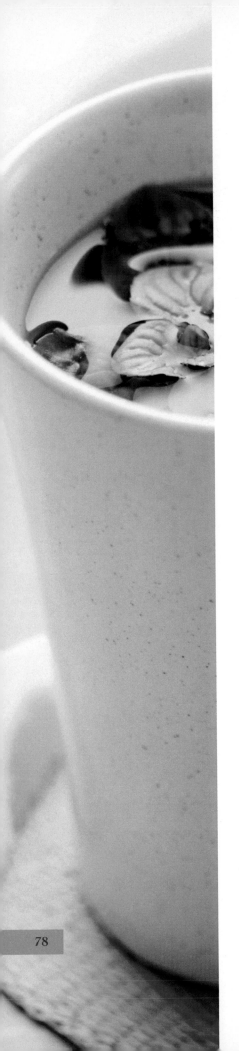

mint & oregano

Mint essential oils and flavoring are used in a large variety of everyday products like toothpaste, chewing gums, alcoholic beverages, herbal teas, ice cream, shampoo, and soap. Of the many different species of mint and hundreds of varieties, spearmint and peppermint are the ones used mainly for their medicinal properties.

Mint has a long history of medicinal use. Recent archaeological discoveries have traced mint's medicinal uses back at least 10,000 years. In ancient Greece and China, mint was made into salves and ointments to treat topical pain because of the cooling and healing effect it brings to the skin.

Peppermint, spearmint, and other mint-family plants are considered some of the most versatile herbs in Chinese medicine. Mint has many well-documented properties. It increases healthy gastric secretions, settles an upset stomach, and alleviates gas. In many countries, fresh mint tea is used after a meal to aid in the digestion of rich foods.

Mint Tea

Place 4 to 5 fresh peppermint leaves in a cup of hot water and allow to steep for 5 minutes. Add natural sweetener such as stevia, honey, or agave to taste, and drink after meals for aiding digestive processes.

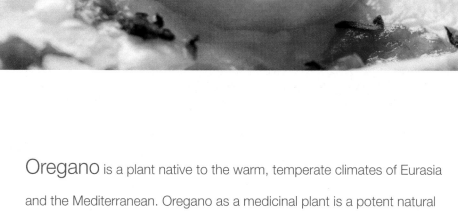

Oregano is a plant native to the warm, temperate climates of Eurasia and the Mediterranean. Oregano as a medicinal plant is a potent natural antibiotic, antifungal, and antiparasitic. These types of problems are common to the large and small intestines and can cause symptoms such as gas bloating, diarrhea, constipation, and IBS (irritable bowel syndrome).

The natural active plant chemicals in oregano, cravacol and thymol, have been shown to be an effective treatment for many types of bacteria, yeast, and parasites commonly found in food and water.

The University of Indiana conducted a research study published in the *Journal of Food Science* that showed concentrated doses of oregano oil to be an effective, natural treatment for E. coli and salmonella bacteria.

Oregano is famous for being the "pizza herb" and is also commonly used in making lasagna and garlic bread.

Spicy Steak Rub

Mix together 2 tablespoons of olive oil, 1 teaspoon of dried oregano, 1/2 teaspoon of red chili flakes, 1/2 teaspoon salt, and 1 tablespoon of freshly ground black pepper. Rub onto a steak before grilling.

The natural active plant chemicals in oregano, cravacol and thymol, have been shown to be an effective natural treatment for many different types of intestinal bacteria, yeast, and parasites.

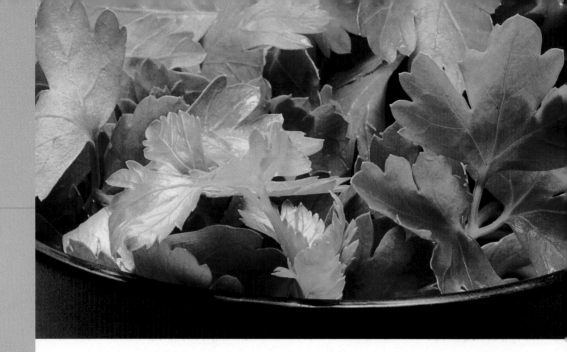

Parsley, cucumber, and lemon make a refreshing and delicious green drink that can be made in a blender. Parsley is very high in natural bioavailable organic iron.

Parsley is a widely cultivated herb and is used in many different types of cuisines around the world. The two most popular types of parsley are curly parsley and Italian flat leaf parsley.

Parsley is native to the Mediterranean region of Southern Europe and has been cultivated for medicinal remedies and as a culinary herb for centuries.

Myristicin is one of the phytochemicals in parsley that help the body eliminate free radical molecules that can do damage to cells and DNA. Parsley is also high in vitamins C, A, and K and is particularly high in easy-to-absorb iron.

Blender Green Drink

Peel and quarter a nice-size cucumber. Cut and wash off the top leaves of 1/2 cup of parsley. Add the juice of 2 fresh lemons. Put everything in a blender, add water and 2 to 3 ice cubes. Blend everything for about 1 minute or until everything is completely blended. For a sweeter flavor, add 1/2 peeled green apple.

parsley & rosemary

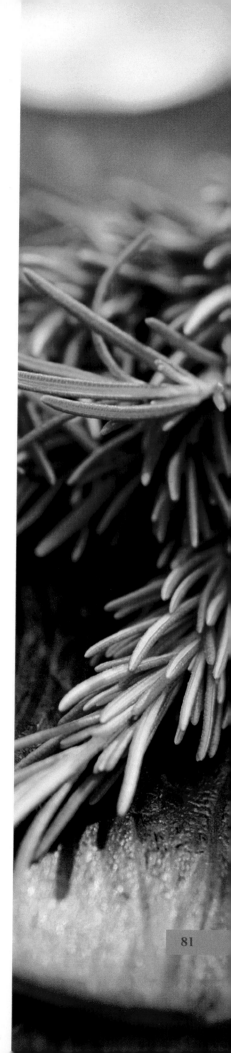

Rosemary is a Mediterranean native that has a distinctive appearance of thick, needle-like, green leaves and pale blue to violet flowers. The Greeks considered it a gift of Aphrodite, the Greek goddess of love and beauty, and brides would wear it as a symbol of their fertility.

Rosemary has been used as a brain tonic in traditional Chinese herbal medicine for thousands of years. It contains phytochemicals that stimulate brain activities and increase brain alertness by increasing blood circulation.

Unlike many other delicate herbs that are added at the end of the cooking process to preserve their flavors, rosemary is best cooked along with food. It pairs well with chicken, lamb, and earthy root vegetables like beets, potatoes, sweet potatoes, and turnips.

Roasted Root Vegetables with Rosemary

Cut 2 cups of beets, red potatoes, sweet potatoes, daikon, or turnips into 1 inch cubes or slices. Add 1 teaspoon of salt and 2 tablespoons of fresh ground pepper. Place in a roasting pan, add 1/2 cup of extra virgin olive oil, and make sure all the vegetables are lightly covered with the oil. Take 2 to 3 sprigs of fresh rosemary, remove the leaves from the stems, and mix in with the vegetables. Bake for 35 to 40 minutes at 375° or until vegetables feel soft. Serve warm. Keeps well in the refrigerator and is great reheated.

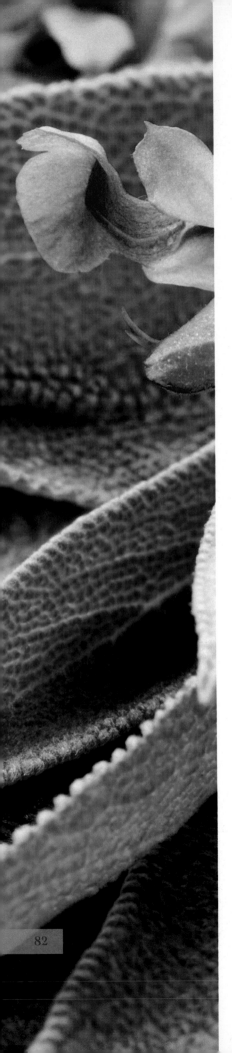

sage & thyme

Sage is a perennial plant with woody stems, grayish leaves, and pretty blue and purple flowers. It is native to the Mediterranean and is now cultivated in many places throughout the world.

It has a long history of medicinal and culinary use and is also used as a popular ornamental garden plant. In England, sage has for generations been listed as one of the essential culinary herbs, along with parsley, rosemary, and thyme.

In traditional Chinese medicine, sage is considered bitter in flavor, slightly cold, and the roots are used medicinally in many herbal formulas to treat irregular menstruation, dysmenorrhea, and amenorrhea.

Sage is best known as an herb used in making stuffing for Christmas and Thanksgiving turkey dinners. The leaves can be used either fresh or dry and also pair well with other herbs. Sage is delicious used with all types of meat and poultry.

Sage Tea Sore Throat Remedy

Take 5-6 (fresh or dried) sage leaves and steep for 3-4 minutes in 2 cups of hot water. Sweeten with honey, if desired. Gargle 2-3 times a day to relieve a sore throat.

Thyme is one of the herbs in the bouquet of the famous French herbal blend called "Herbes de Provence" and is used in cheeses and liqueurs to add flavor and aroma.

Thyme is a very aromatic, perennial, low-growing plant with flowers ranging in color from white to lilac and purple. Thyme loves warm, sunny climates and is native to southern Europe.

The essential oil extracted from the thyme leaves has been used as a natural antibiotic. Before the advent of modern antibiotics, oil of thyme was used to medicate bandages and then placed on wounds. It has been used as a medicinal tea for sore throats. Studies have shown that thymol, the active photochemical found in thyme, inhibits the growth of fungus and certain types of bacteria. Many commercially produced mouthwashes, such as Listerine, contain oil of eucalyptus and essential oil of thyme.

This herb adds a distinctive aromatic flavoring to sauces, stews, stuffing, meats, and many types of savory dishes. Thyme is one of the herbs in the bouquet of the famous French herbal blend called *Herbes de Provence,* and is used in cheeses and liqueurs to add flavor and aroma.

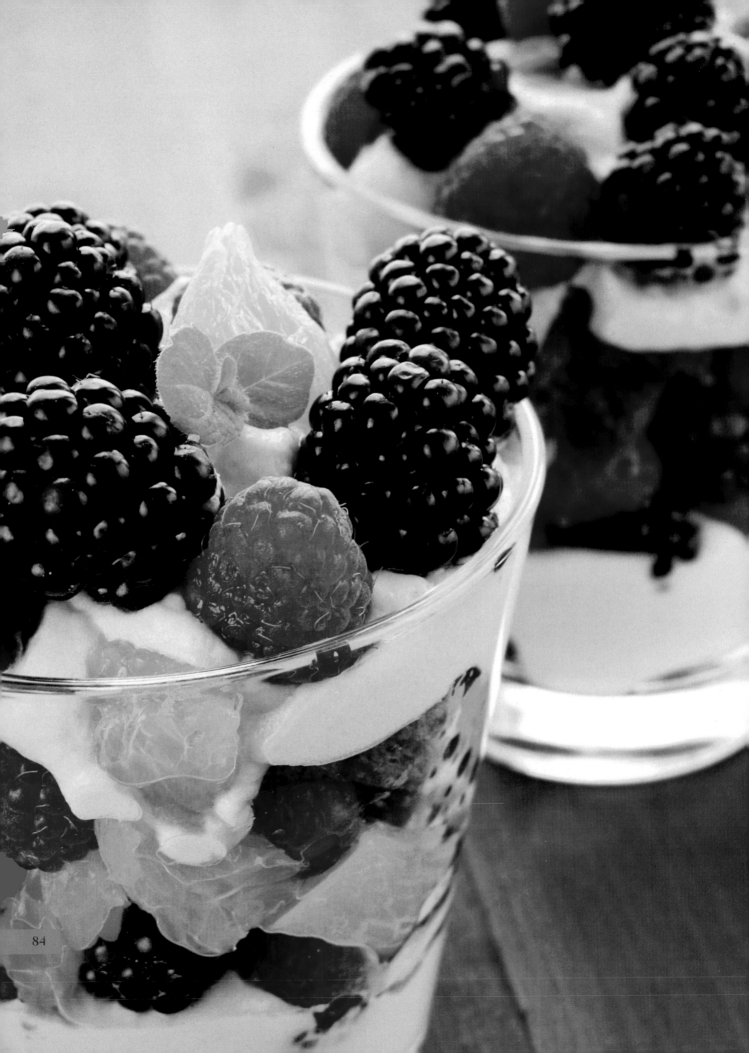

Eating with Intention and Awareness

Plants have been used for thousand of years for cooking as well as medicines. From ancient cultures come elaborate cuisines along with the knowledge of how foods and herbs can cure and heal the body. So many plants have natural medicinal properties, and the ones I have chosen to write about have perhaps the most concentrated medicinal properties and may also be the least known about.

The scientifically proven medicinal compounds found in fruits, flowers, spices, herbs, and vegetables can help to naturally change our health and vitality.

Fresh organic fruits and vegetables not only are delicious but offer us an infinite variety of colors, textures, aromas, and tastes. They also provide extra excitement and enjoyment to any simple salads, fresh and baked fruit desserts, and all savory dishes.

Healthy lifestyle changes such as diet and exercise have been proven to reverse disease processes as well as become our best preventative medicine. With chronic and serious diseases on the rise in this country, we must make our health, and the health of our family and friends, a priority.

"Eating a high-nutrient diet actually makes you more satisfied with less food, and actually gives the ability to enjoy food more without overeating."

— Dr. Joel Fuhrman

Joel Fuhrman, M.D. is an expert in the field of nutrition.

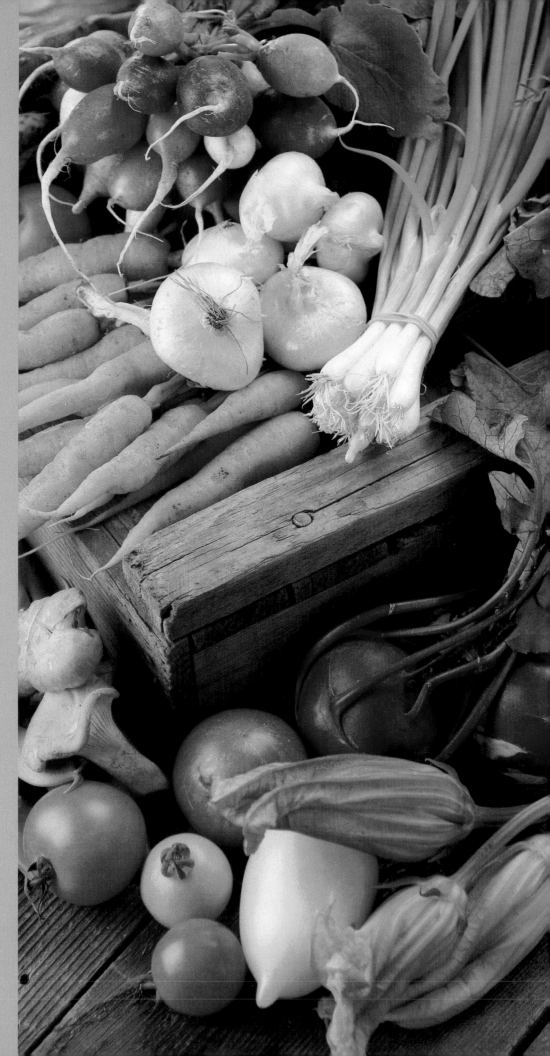

"If we are creating ourselves all the time, then it is never too late to begin creating the bodies we want instead of the ones we mistakenly assume we are stuck with."

— Deepak Chopra, M.D.

Deepak Chopra is founder of the Chopra Center and author of 22 *New York Times* best-sellers.